HEALTHY GUT

THE

DIGESTIVE

MIRACLE

The Proven 7 Day Detox Low
Carb Keto Gut Healing
Cookbook For a Better You

KIERAN PARKER

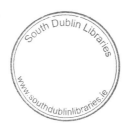

from the Publisher. All additional right reserved.

The information in the following pages is broadly considered to be a truthful and accurate account of facts and as such any inattention, use or misuse of the information in question by the reader will render any resulting actions solely under their purview. There are no scenarios in which the publisher or the original author of this work can be in any fashion deemed liable for any hardship or damages that may befall them after undertaking information described herein.

Additionally, the information in the following pages is intended only for informational purposes and should thus be thought of as universal. As befitting its nature, it is presented without assurance regarding its prolonged validity or interim quality. Trademarks that are mentioned are done without written consent and can in no way be considered an endorsement from the trademark holder.

Table of Contents

PART I

The sirtfood diet is one of the latest diet patterns that has garnered quite the attention. The idea was brought to the market by two nutritionists Glen Matten and Aidan Goggins. The main idea of the diet revolves around sirtuins, which are basically a group of 7 proteins that are responsible for the functioning and regulation of lifespan, inflammation, and metabolism (Sergiy Libert, 2013).

Chapter 1: Health Benefits of the Diet

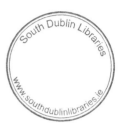

The benefits are vast. This includes loss in weight, better skin quality, gain in muscle mass in the areas that are very much required, increased metabolic rate, feeling of fullness without having to eat much (this is the power of the foods actually), suppressing the appetite, and leading a better and confident life. This specifically includes an increase in the memory, supporting the body to control blood sugar and blood cholesterol level in a much-advanced way, and wiping out the damage caused by the free radicals and thus preventing them from having adverse impacts on the cells that might lead to other diseases like cancer.

The consumption of these foods, along with the drinks, has a number of observational shreds of evidence that link the sirtfoods with the reducing hazards of several chronic diseases. This diet is notably suited as an anti-aging scheme. Sirtfoods have the ability to satiate the appetite in a natural way and increase the functioning of the muscle. These two points are enough to find a solution that can ultimately help us to achieve a healthy weight. In addition to this, the health-improving impact of these compounds is powerful in comparison to the drugs that are prescribed in order to prevent several chronic diseases like that of diabetes, heart problems, Alzheimer's, etc.

A pilot study was conducted on a total of 39 participants. At the end of the first week, the participants had an increase in muscle mass and also lost 7 pounds on average. Research has proven that in this initial week, the weight loss that is witnessed is mostly from water, glycogen, and muscle, and only one-third of it is from fat (Manfred J. Müller, 2016). The major sirtfoods include red wine, kale, soy, strawberries, matcha green tea, extra virgin olive oil, walnuts, buckwheat, capers, lovage, coffee, dark chocolate, Medjool dates, turmeric, red chicory, parsley, onions, arugula, and blueberries (Kathrin Pallauf, 2013).

Chapter 2: Sirtfood Juice Recipes

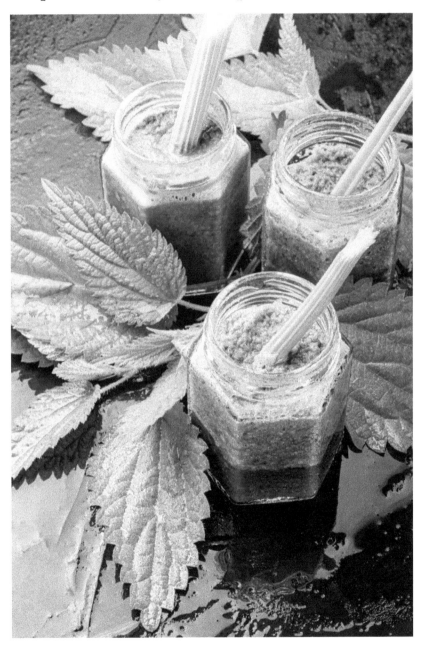

Green Juice

Total Prep & Cooking Time: Five minutes

Yields: 1 serving

Nutrition Facts: Calories: 182.3 | Carbs: 42.9g | Protein: 6g | Fat: 1.5g | Fiber: 12.7g

Ingredients:

- Half a green apple
- Two sticks of celery
- Five grams of parsley
- Thirty grams of rocket
- Seventy-five grams of kale
- Half a teaspoon of matcha green tea
- Juice of half a lemon
- One cm of ginger

Method:

1. Juice the kale, rocket, celery sticks, green apple, and parsley in a juicer.

2. Add the lemon juice into the green juice by squeezing it with your hand.

3. Take a glass and pour a little amount of the green juice into it. Add the matcha green tea and stir it in. Then, pour the remaining green juice into the glass and stir to combine everything properly.

4. You can choose to save it for later or drink it straight away.

Blueberry Kale Smoothie

Total Prep & Cooking Time: Five minutes

Yields: 1 serving

Nutrition Facts: Calories: 240 | Carbs: 37.9g | Protein: 17.2g | Fat: 3.6g | Fiber: 7g

Ingredients:

- Half a cup each of
  - Plain low-fat yogurt
  - Blueberries (frozen or fresh)
  - Kale, chopped
- Half a banana
- Half a teaspoon of cinnamon powder
- One tablespoon of flaxseed meal
- One scoop of protein powder
- Half a cup of water (optional)
- Two handfuls of ice (you can add more if you like)

Method:

1. Take a high-speed blender and add all the ingredients in it.

2. Blend everything together until you get a smooth puree.

3. Pour the blueberry kale smoothie in a glass and serve cold.

Tropical Kale Smoothie

Total Prep & Cooking Time: 10 minutes

Yields: 2 servings

Nutrition Facts: Calories: 187 | Carbs: 46.8g | Protein: 3.5g | Fat: 0.5g | Fiber: 4.7g

Ingredients:

- Half a cup to one cup of orange juice (about 120 ml to 240 ml)
- One banana, chopped (use frozen banana, is possible)
- Two cups of pineapple (about 330 grams), chopped (use frozen pineapple if possible)
- One and a half cups of kale (around 90 grams), chopped

Method:

1. Add the chopped bananas, pineapple, kale, and orange juice into a blender and blend everything together until you get a smooth puree.

2. You can add more orange juice if you need to attain a smoothie consistency. The amount of frozen fruit used directly affects the consistency of the smoothie.

3. Pour the smoothie equally into two glasses and serve cold.

Strawberry Oatmeal Smoothie

Total Prep & Cooking Time: 5 minutes

Yields: 2 servings

Nutrition Facts: Calories: 236.1 | Carbs: 44.9g | Protein: 7.6g | Fat: 3.7g | Fiber: 5.9g

Ingredients:

- Half a tsp. of vanilla extract
- Fourteen frozen strawberries
- One banana (cut into chunks)
- Half a cup of rolled oats
- One cup of soy milk
- One and a half tsps. of white sugar

Method:

1. Take a blender. Add the strawberries, banana, oats, and soy milk.
2. Then add sugar and vanilla extract.
3. Blend until the texture becomes smooth.
4. Then pour it into a glass and serve.

Chapter 3: Main Course Recipes for Sirtfood Diet

Green Juice Salad

Total Prep & Cooking Time: Ten minutes

Yields: 1 serving

Nutrition Facts: Calories: 199 | Carbs: 27g | Protein: 10g | Fat: 8.2g | Fiber: 9.2g

Ingredients:

- Six walnuts, halved
- Half of a green apple, sliced
- Two sticks of celery, sliced
- One tablespoon each of
  - Parsley
  - Olive oil
- One handful of rocket
- Two handfuls of kale, sliced
- One cm of ginger, grated
- Juice of half a lemon
- Salt and pepper to taste

Method:

1. To make the dressing, add the olive oil, ginger, lemon juice, salt, and pepper in a jam jar. Shake the jar to combine everything together.

2. Keep the sliced kale in a large bowl and add the dressing over it. Massage the dressing for about a minute to mix it with the kale properly.

3. Lastly, add the remaining ingredients (walnuts, sliced green apple, celery sticks, parsley, and rocket) into the bowl and combine everything thoroughly.

King Prawns and Buckwheat Noodles

Total Prep & Cooking Time: Twenty minutes

Yields: 4 servings

Nutrition Facts: Calories: 496 | Carbs: 53.2g | Protein: 22.2g | Fat: 17.6g | Fiber: 4.8g

Ingredients:

- 600 grams of king prawn
- 300 grams of soba or buckwheat noodles (using 100 percent buckwheat is recommended)
- One bird's eye chili, membranes, and seeds eliminated and finely chopped (and more according to taste)
- Three cloves of garlic, finely chopped or grated
- Three cm of ginger, grated
- 100 grams of green beans, chopped
- 100 grams of kale, roughly chopped
- Two celery sticks, sliced
- One red onion, thinly sliced
- Two tablespoons each of
  - Parsley, finely chopped (or lovage, if you have it)
  - Soy sauce or tamari (and extra for serving)
  - Extra virgin olive oil

Method:

1. Boil the buckwheat noodles for three to five minutes or until they are cooked according to your liking. Drain the water and then rinse the noodles in cold water. Drizzle some olive oil on the top and mix it with the noodles. Keep this mixture aside.

2. Prepare the remaining ingredients while the noodles are boiling.

3. Place a large frying pan or a wok over low heat and add a little olive oil into it. Then add the celery and red onions and fry them for about three minutes so that they get soft.

4. Then add the green beans and kale and increase the heat to medium-high. Fry them for about three minutes.

5. Decrease the heat again and then add the prawns, chili, ginger, and garlic into the pan. Fry for another two to three minutes so that the prawns get hot all the way through.

6. Lastly, add in the buckwheat noodles, soy sauce/tamari, and cook it for another minute so that the noodles get warm again.

7. Sprinkle some chopped parsley on the top as a garnish and serve hot.

Red Onion Dhal and Buckwheat

Total Prep & Cooking Time: Thirty minutes

Yields: 4 servings

Nutrition Facts: Calories: 154 | Carbs: 9g | Protein: 19g | Fat: 2g | Fiber: 12g

Ingredients:

- 160 grams of buckwheat or brown rice
- 100 grams of kale (spinach would also be a good alternative)
- 200 ml of water
- 400 ml of coconut milk
- 160 grams of red lentils
- Two teaspoons each of
  - Garam masala
  - Turmeric
- One bird's eye chili, deseeded and finely chopped (plus more if you want it extra hot)
- Two cms of ginger, grated
- Three cloves of garlic, crushed or grated
- One red onion (small), sliced
- One tablespoon of olive oil

Method:

1. Take a large, deep saucepan and add the olive oil in it. Add the sliced onion and cook it on low heat with the lid closed for about five minutes so that they get softened.

2. Add the chili, ginger, and garlic and cook it for another minute.

3. Add a splash of water along with the garam masala and turmeric and cook for another minute.

4. Next add the coconut milk, red lentils along with 200 ml of water. You can do this by filling the can of coconut milk halfway with water and adding it into the saucepan.

5. Combine everything together properly and let it cook over low heat for about twenty minutes. Keep the lid on and keep stirring occasionally. If the dhal starts to stick to the pan, add a little more water to it.

6. Add the kale after twenty minutes and stir properly and put the lid back on. Let it cook for another five minutes. (If you're using spinach instead, cook for an additional one to two minutes)

7. Add the buckwheat in a medium-sized saucepan about fifteen minutes before the curry is cooked.

8. Add lots of boiling water into the buckwheat and boil the water again—Cook for about ten minutes. If you prefer softer buckwheat, you can cook it for a little longer.

9. Drain the buckwheat using a sieve and serve along with the dhal.

Chicken Curry

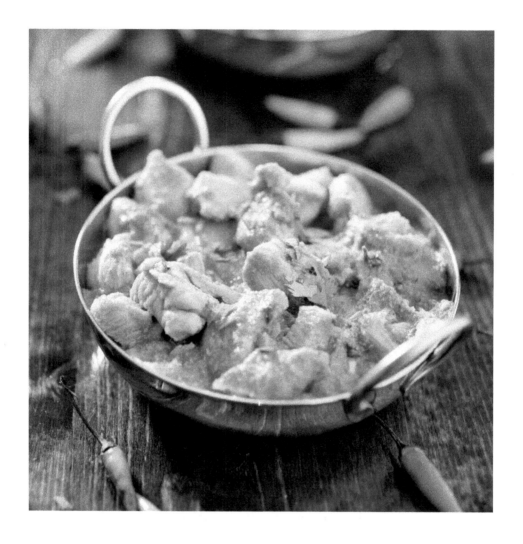

Total Prep & Cooking Time: 45 minutes

Yields: 4 servings

Nutrition Facts: Calories: 243 | Carbs: 7.5g | Protein: 28g | Fat: 11g | Fiber: 1.5g

Ingredients:

- 200 grams of buckwheat (you can also use basmati rice or brown rice)
- One 400ml tin of coconut milk
- Eight skinless and boneless chicken thighs, sliced into bite-sized chunks (you can also use four chicken breasts)
- One tablespoon of olive oil
- Six cardamom pods (optional)
- One cinnamon stick (optional)
- Two teaspoons each of
  - Ground turmeric
  - Ground cumin
  - Garam masala
- Two cm. of fresh ginger, peeled and coarsely chopped
- Three cloves of garlic, roughly chopped
- One red onion, roughly chopped
- Two tablespoons of freshly chopped coriander (and more for garnishing)

Method:

1. Add the ginger, garlic, and onions in a food processor and blitz to get a paste. You can also use a hand blender to make the paste. If you have neither, just finely chop the three ingredients and continue the following steps.

2. Add the turmeric powder, cumin, and garam masala into the paste and combine them together. Keep the paste aside.

3. Take a wide, deep pan (preferably a non-stick pan) and add one tablespoon of olive oil into it. Heat it over high heat for about a minute and then add the pieces of boneless chicken thighs. Increase the heat and stir-fry the chicken thighs for about two minutes. Then, reduce the heat and add the curry paste. Let the chicken cook in the curry paste for about three minutes and then pour half of the coconut milk (about 200ml) into it. You can also add the cardamom and cinnamon if you're using them.

4. Let it boil for some time and then reduce the heat and let it simmer for thirty minutes. The curry sauce will get thick and delicious.

5. You can add a splash of coconut milk if your curry sauce begins to get dry. You might not need to add extra coconut milk at all, but you can add it if you want a slightly more saucy curry.

6. Prepare your side dishes and other accompaniments (buckwheat or rice) while the curry is cooking.

7. Add the chopped coriander as a garnish when the curry is ready and serve immediately with the buckwheat or rice.

Chickpea Stew With Baked Potatoes

Total Prep & Cooking Time: One hour and ten minutes

Yields: 4 to 6 servings

Nutrition Facts: Calories: 348.3 | Carbs: 41.2g | Protein: 7.2g | Fat: 16.5g | Fiber: 5.3g

Ingredients:

- Two yellow peppers, chopped into bite-sized pieces (you can also use other colored bell peppers)
- Two 400-grams tins each of
    - Chickpeas (you can also use kidney beans) (don't drain the water if you prefer including it)
    - Chopped tomatoes
- Two cm. of ginger, grated
- Four cloves of garlic, crushed or grated
- Two red onions, finely chopped
- Four to six potatoes, prickled all over
- Two tablespoons each of
    - Turmeric
    - Cumin seeds
    - Olive oil
    - Unsweetened cocoa powder (or cacao, if you want)
    - Parsley (and extra for garnishing)
- Half a teaspoon to two teaspoons of chili flakes (you can add according to how hot you like things)
- A splash of water
- Side salad (optional)
- Salt and pepper according to your taste (optional)

Method:

1. Preheat your oven to 200 degrees Celsius.

2. In the meantime, prepare all the other ingredients.

3. Place your baking potatoes in the oven when it gets hot enough and allow it to cook for an hour so that they are cooked according to your preference. You can also use your regular method to bake the potatoes if it's different from this method.

4. When the potatoes are cooking in the oven, place a large wide saucepan over low heat and add the olive oil along with the chopped red onion into it. Keep the lid on and let the onions cook for five minutes. The onions should turn soft but shouldn't turn brown.

5. Take the lid off and add the chili, cumin, ginger, and garlic into the saucepan. Let it cook on low heat for another minute and then add the turmeric along with a tiny splash of water and cook it for a further minute. Make sure that the pan does not get too dry.

6. Then, add in the yellow pepper, canned chickpeas (along with the chickpea liquid), cacao or cocoa powder, and chopped tomatoes. Bring the mixture to a boil and then let it simmer on low heat for about forty-five minutes so that the sauce gets thick and unctuous (make sure that it doesn't burn). The stew and the potatoes should complete cooking at roughly the same time.

7. Finally, add some salt and pepper as per your taste along with the parsley and stir them in the stew.

8. You can add the stew on top of the baked potatoes and serve. You can also serve the stew with a simple side salad.

Blueberry Pancakes

Total Prep & Cooking Time: 25 minutes

Yields: 2 servings

Nutrition Facts: Calories: 84 | Carbs: 11g | Protein: 2.3g | Fat: 3.5g | Fiber: 0g

Ingredients:

- 225 grams of blueberries
- 150 grams of rolled oats
- Six eggs
- Six bananas
- One-fourth of a teaspoon of salt
- Two teaspoons of baking powder

Method:

1. Add the rolled oats in a high-speed blender and pulse it for about a minute or so to get the oat flour. Before adding the oats to the blender, make sure that it is very dry. Otherwise, your oat flour will turn soggy.

2. Then, add the eggs and bananas along with the salt and baking soda into the blender and blend them together for another two minutes until you get a smooth batter.

3. Take a large bowl and transfer the mixture into it. Then add the blueberries and fold them into the mixture. Let it rest for about ten minutes to allow the baking powder to activate.

4. To make the pancakes, place a frying pan on medium-high heat and add a dollop of butter into it. The butter will help to make your pancakes really crispy and delicious.

5. Add a few spoonfuls of the blueberry pancake batter into the frying pan and cook it until the bottom side turns golden. Once the bottom turns golden, toss the pancake and fry the other side.

6. Serve them hot and enjoy.

Sirtfood Bites

Total Prep & Cooking Time: 1 hour + 15 minutes

Yields: 15-20 bites

Nutrition Facts: Calories: 58.1 | Carbs: 10.1g | Protein: 0.9g | Fat: 2.3g | Fiber: 1.2g

Ingredients:

- One tablespoon each of
  - Extra virgin olive oil
  - Ground turmeric
  - Cocoa powder
- Nine ounces of Medjool dates, pitted (about 250 grams)
- One ounce (about thirty grams) of dark chocolate (85% cocoa solids), break them into pieces (you can also use one-fourth of a cup of cocoa nibs)
- One teaspoon of vanilla extract (you can also take the scraped seeds of one vanilla pod)
- One cup of walnuts (about 120 grams)
- One to two tablespoons of water

Method:

1. Add the chocolate and walnuts in a food processor and blitz them until you get a fine powder.

2. Add the Medjool dates, cocoa powder, ground turmeric, extra-virgin olive oil, and vanilla extract into the food processor and blend them together until the mixture forms a ball. Depending on the consistency of the mixture, you can choose to add or skip the water. Make sure that the mixture is not too sticky.

3. Make bite-sized balls from the mixture using your hands and keep them in the refrigerator in an airtight container. Refrigerate them for at least an hour before consuming them.

4. To get a finish of your liking, you can roll the balls in some more dried coconut or cocoa. You can store the balls in the refrigerator for up to a week.

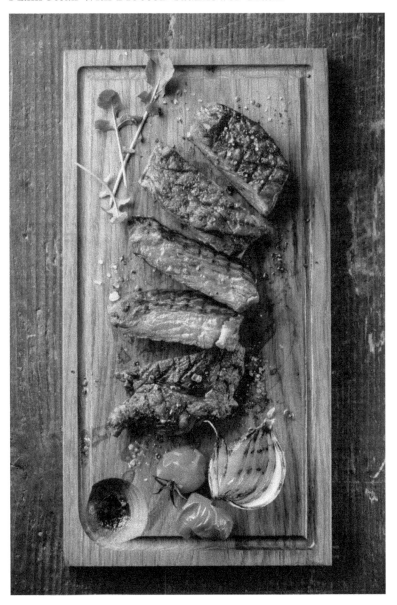

Total Prep & Cooking Time: 55 minutes

Yields: 4 servings

Nutrition Facts: Calories: 839 | Carbs: 8g | Protein: 43g | Fat: 70g | Fiber: 3g

Ingredients:

- Two tablespoons of olive oil
- Twenty ounces of flank steak
- One-fourth teaspoon salt
- Four ounces of divided shredded cheese
- Half cup of heavy whipping cream
- Eight ounces of cauliflower
- Eight ounces of broccoli
- Salt and pepper

For the pepper sauce,

- One tablespoon soy sauce
- One and a half cups of heavy whipping cream
- Half teaspoon ground black pepper

For the garnishing,

- Two tablespoons of freshly chopped parsley

Method:

1. At first, you have to preheat your oven to four hundred degrees Fahrenheit. Then you need to apply butter on a baking dish (eight by eight inches).

2. Then you have to clean and then trim the cauliflower and broccoli. Then you need to cut them into florets, and their stem needs to be sliced.

3. Then you have to boil the broccoli and cauliflower for about five minutes in salted water.

4. After boiling, you need to drain out all the water and keep the vegetables aside. Then you have to take a saucepan over medium heat and add half portion of the shredded cheese, heavy cream, and salt. Then you need to whisk them together until the cheese gets melted. Then you have to add the cauliflower and the broccoli and mix them in.

5. Place the cauliflower and broccoli mixture in a baking dish. Then you have to take the rest half portion of the cheese and add—Bake for about twenty minutes in the oven.

6. Season with salt and pepper on both sides of the meat.

7. Then you have to take a large frying pan over medium-high heat and fry the meat for about four to five minutes on each side.

8. After that, take a cutting board and place the meat on it. Then you have to leave the meat for about ten to fifteen minutes before you start to slice it.

9. Take the frying pan, and in it, you need to pour soy sauce, cream, and pepper. Then you have to bring it to a boil and allow the sauce to simmer until the sauce becomes creamy in texture. Then you need to taste it and then season it with some more salt and pepper according to your taste.

Kale Celery Salad

Total Prep & Cooking Time: 15 minutes

Yields: 4 servings

Nutrition Facts: 196 | Carbs: 20g | Protein: 5.7g | Fat: 11.5g | Fiber: 4.8g

Ingredients:

- Half a cup of crumbled feta cheese
- Half a cup of chopped and toasted walnuts
- One wedge lemon
- One red apple, crisp
- Two celery stalks
- Eight dates, pitted dried
- Four cups of washed and dried baby kale (stemmed)

For the dressing,

- Three tbsps. olive oil
- One tsp. maple syrup (or you can use any other sweetener as per your preference)
- Four tsps. balsamic vinegar
- Freshly ground salt and black pepper

Method:

1. At first, you have to take a platter or a wide serving bowl. Then you need to place the baby kale in it.

2. Cut the dates into very thin slices, lengthwise. Then you need to place it in another small bowl.

3. After that, you have to peel the celery and then cut them into halves, lengthwise.

4. Then you need to take your knife, hold it in a diagonal angle, and then cut the celery into thin pieces (approximately one to two inches each). Add these pieces to the dates.

5. Then you have to cut the sides off the apple. You need to cut very thin slices from those pieces.

6. Over the apple slices, you need to put some lemon juice to prevent them from browning.

7. For preparing the dressing, you have to take a small bowl, add maple syrup, olive oil, and vinegar. Then you need to whisk them together.

8. Once done, you have to season with freshly ground pepper and two pinches of salt.

9. Before serving, you need to take most of the dressing and pour it over the salad. Then you have to toss nicely so that they get combined. Then you need to pour the rest of the portion of the dressing over the dates and celery.

10. On the top, you have to add the date mixture, feta cheese, apple slices, and walnuts.

Buckwheat Stir Fry

Total Prep & Cooking Time: 28 minutes

Yields: 8 servings

Nutrition Facts: Calories: 258 | Carbs: 35.1g | Protein: 6.8g | Fat: 11.9g | Fiber: 2g

Ingredients:

For the buckwheat,

- Three cups of water
- One and a half cups of uncooked roasted buckwheat groats
- Pinch of salt

For the stir fry,

- Half a cup of finely chopped basil
- Half a cup of finely chopped parsley
- One teaspoon salt
- Four tablespoons of divided red palm oil or coconut oil
- Two cups of drained and chopped marinated artichoke hearts
- Four large bell peppers (sliced into strips)
- Four large minced cloves of garlic
- One bunch of finely chopped kale (ribs removed)

Method:

For making the buckwheat,

1. In a medium-sized pot, pour the buckwheat. Then rinse with cold water and drain the water. Repeat this process for about two to three times.

2. Then add three cups of water to it and also add a pinch of salt. Cover the pot and bring it to a boil.

3. Reduce the heat to low and then cook for about fifteen minutes. Keep the lid on and remove the pot from the heat.

4. Leave it for three minutes and then fluff with a fork.

For making the stir fry,

1. At first, you have to take a ceramic non-stick wok and preheat over medium heat. Then you need to add one tablespoon of oil and coat it. Then you have to add garlic and then sauté for about ten seconds. Then you need to add kale and then add one-fourth teaspoon of salt. Then you need to sauté it accompanied by occasional stirring, until it shrinks in half. Then you have to transfer it to a medium-sized bowl.

2. Then again return to the wok, turn the heat on high, and pour one tablespoon of oil. You need to add one-fourth teaspoon salt and pepper. Then you have to sauté it until it turns golden brown in color. Once done, you need to place it in the bowl containing kale.

3. Then you have to reduce the heat to low, and you need to add two tablespoons of oil. Add the cooked buckwheat and stir it nicely so that it gets coated in the oil. Then after turning off the heat, you need to add the kale and peppers, basil, parsley, artichoke hearts, and half teaspoon salt. Gently stir and serve it hot.

Kale Omelet

Total Prep & Cooking Time: 10 minutes

Yields: 1 serving

Nutrition Facts: Calories: 339 | Carbs: 8.6g | Protein: 15g | Fat: 28.1g | Fiber: 4.4g

Ingredients:

- One-fourth sliced avocado
- Pinch of red pepper (crushed)
- One tsp. sunflower seeds (unsalted)
- One tbsp. of freshly chopped cilantro
- One tbsp. lime juice
- One cup of chopped kale
- Two tsps. of extra-virgin olive oil
- One tsp. of low-fat milk
- Two eggs
- Salt

Method:

1. At first, take a small bowl and pour milk. Then you have to add the eggs and salt to it. Beat the mixture thoroughly. Then take a small non-stick

skillet over medium heat, and add one tsp. of oil and heat it. Then add the egg mixture and cook for about one to two minutes, until the time you notice that the center is still a bit runny, but the bottom has become set. Then you need to flip the omelet and cook the other side for another thirty seconds until it is set too. One done, transfer the omelet to a plate.

2. Toss the kale with one tsp. of oil, sunflower seeds, cilantro, lime juice, salt, and crushed red pepper in another bowl. Then return to the omelet on the plate and top it off with avocado and the kale salad.

Tuna Rocket Salad

Total Prep & Cooking Time: 20 minutes

Yields: 4 servings

Nutrition Facts: Calories: 321 | Carbs: 20g | Protein: 33g | Fat: 12g | Fiber: 9.5g

Ingredients:

- Twelve leaves of basil (fresh)
- Two bunches of washed and dried rocket (trimmed)
- One and a half tbsps. of olive oil
- Freshly ground black pepper and salt
- Sixty grams of kalamata olives cut into halves, lengthwise (drained pitted)
- One thinly sliced and halved red onion
- Two coarsely chopped ripe tomatoes
- Four hundred grams of rinsed and drained cannellini beans
- Four hundred grams of drained tuna
- 2 cm cubes of one multigrain bread roll

Method:

1. At first, you need to preheat your oven to 200 degrees Celsius.

2. After that, take a baking tray and line it with a foil.

3. Then you have to spread the cubes of bread over the baking tray evenly.

4. Put the baking tray inside the oven and cook it for about ten minutes until it turns golden in color.

5. In the meantime, you have to take a large bowl and add the olives, onions, tomatoes, cannellini beans, and tuna. Then you need to season it with pepper and salt. Add some oil and then toss for smooth combining.

6. Your next step is to add the basil leaves, croutons, and the rocket. Then you need to toss gently to combine. After that, you can divide the salad into the serving bowls and serve.

Turmeric Baked Salmon

Total Prep & Cooking Time: 30 minutes

Yields: 4 servings

Nutrition Facts: Calories: 448 | Carbs: 2g | Protein: 34g | Fat: 33g | Fiber: 0.2g

Ingredients:

- One ripe yellow lemon
- Half a teaspoon of salt
- One teaspoon turmeric
- One tablespoon of dried thyme
- Half a cup of frozen, salted butter (you may require some more for greasing the pan)
- Four fresh one and a half inches thick salmon fillets (skin-on)

Method:

1. At first, you need to preheat your oven to 400 degrees Fahrenheit. Then with a thin layer of butter, you need to grease the bottom of the baking sheet. Rinse the salmon fillets and pat them dry. Then you have to place the salmon fillets on the buttered baking dish keeping the skin side down.

2. Take the lemons and cut them into four round slices. Remove the seeds and then cut each slice into two halves. Then you will have eight pieces.

3. Take a small dish and combine turmeric, dried thyme, and salt. Then you need to mix them well until they are nicely combined. On the top of the salmon fillets, you need to evenly sprinkle the spice mixture.

4. Place two lemon slices over each salmon fillet.

5. After that, you need to grate the cold butter on the top of the salmon fillets evenly. Allow the butter to meltdown and form a delicious sauce.

6. Then you have to cover the pan with parchment or aluminum foil. Put it inside the oven and cook for about fifteen to twenty minutes according to your desire. The cooking time is dependent on the thickness of the salmon fillets. You can check whether it is done or not by cutting into the center.

7. Once done, remove it from the oven and then uncover it. The butter sauce needs to be spooned over from the tray.

8. Top it off with fresh mint and serve.

Chapter 4: One-Week Meal Plan

Day 1

8 AM – Green Juice

12 PM - Blueberry Kale Smoothie

4 PM – Tropical Kale Smoothie

8 PM – Turmeric Baked Salmon

Day 2

8 AM – Tropical Kale Smoothie

12 PM – Green Juice

4 PM – Strawberry Oatmeal Smoothie

8 PM – King Prawns and Buckwheat Noodles

Day 3

8 AM – Strawberry Oatmeal Smoothie

12 PM – Tropical Kale Smoothie

4 PM – Green Juice

8 PM – Buckwheat Stir Fry

Day 4

8 AM – Blueberry Kale Smoothie

12 PM – Green Juice

4 PM – Green Juice Salad

8 PM – Tuna Rocket Salad

Day 5

8 AM – Green Juice

12 PM – Tropical Kale Smoothie

4 PM – Sirtfood Bites

8 PM – Chicken Curry

Day 6

8 AM – Strawberry Oatmeal Smoothie

12 PM – Green Juice

4 PM – Kale Celery Salad

8 PM – Flank Steak with Broccoli Cauliflower Gratin

Day 7

8 AM – Tropical Kale Smoothie

12 PM – Blueberry Kale Smoothie

4 PM – Kale Omelet

8 PM – Chickpea Stew with Baked Potatoes

PART II

In this chapter, we are going to study the details of the reset diet and what recipes you can make.

Chapter 1: How to Reset Your Body?

Created by a celebrity trainer, Harley Pasternak, the body reset diet is a famous fifteen-day eating pattern that aims to jump-start weight loss. According to Pasternak, if you experience rapid loss in weight early in a diet, you will feel more motivated to stick to that diet plan. This theory is even supported by a few scientific studies (Alice A Gibson, 2017).

The body reset diet claims to help in weight loss with light exercise and low-calorie diet plans for fifteen days. The diet is divided into 3 phases of five days each. Each phase had a particular pattern of diet and exercise routine. You need to consume food five times every day, starting from the first phase, which mostly consists of smoothies and progressing to more solid foods in the second and third phases.

The three phases of the body reset diet are:

- **Phase One** – During this stage, you are required to consume only two snacks every day and drink smoothies for breakfast, lunch, and dinner. In the case of exercise, you have to walk at least ten thousand steps per day.

- **Phase Two** – During this phase, you can eat two snacks each day, consume solid food only once, and have to replace any two meals of the day with smoothies. In case of exercise, apart from walking ten thousand steps every day, on three of the days, you also have to finish five minutes of resistance training with the help of four separate exercises.

- **Phase Three** – You can consume two snacks every day, but you have to eat two low-calorie meals and replace one of your meals with a smoothie. For exercise, you are required to walk ten thousand steps. Apart from that, you also have to finish five minutes of resistance training with the help of four separate exercises each day.

After you have finished the standard fifteen-day diet requirements, you have to keep following the meal plan you followed in the third phase. However, during this time, you are allowed to have two "free meals" twice a week in which you can consume anything you want. These "free meals" are meant as a reward so that you can avoid feeling deprived. According to Pasternak, depriving yourself of a particular food continuously can result in binge eating (Nawal Alajmi, 2016).

There is no official endpoint of the diet after the first fifteen days for losing and maintaining weight. Pasternak suggests that the habits and routines formed over fifteen days should be maintained for a lifetime.

Chapter 2: Science Behind Metabolism Reset

Several people take on a "cleanse" or "detox" diet every year to lose the extra holiday weight or simply start following healthy habits. However, some fat diet plans are often a bit overwhelming. For example, it requires a tremendous amount of self-discipline to drink only juices. Moreover, even after finishing a grueling detox diet plan, you might just go back to eating foods that are bad for you because of those days of deprivation. New studies issued in the *Medicine & Science in Sports & Exercise* shows that low-calorie diets may result in binge eating, which is not the right method for lasting weight loss.

Another research conducted by the researchers at Loughborough University showed that healthy, college-aged women who followed a calorie-restricted diet consumed an extra three hundred calories at dinner as compared to the control group who consumed three standard meals. They revealed that it was because they had lower levels of peptide YY (represses appetite) and higher levels of ghrelin (makes you hungry). They are most likely to go hog wild when you are feeling ravenous, and it's finally time to eat (Nawal Alajmi K. D.-O., 2016).

Another research published in *Cognitive Neuroscience* studied the brains of chronic dieters. They revealed that there was a weaker connection between the two regions of the brain in people who had a higher percentage of body fat. They showed that they might have an increased risk of getting obese because it's harder for them to set their temptations aside (Pin-Hao Andy Chen, 2016).

A few other studies, however, also revealed that you could increase your self-control through practice. Self-control, similar to any other kind of strength, also requires time to develop. However, you can consider focusing on a diet plan that can help you "reset" instead of putting all your efforts into developing your self-control to get healthy.

A reset is considered as a new start – one that can get your metabolism and your liver in good shape. The liver is the biggest solid organ of your body, and it's mainly responsible for removing toxins that can harm your health and well-being by polluting your system. Toxins keep accumulating in your body all the time, and even though it's the liver's job to handle this, it can sometimes get behind schedule, which can result in inflammation. It causes a lot of strain on your metabolism and results in weight gain, particularly around the abdomen. The best method to alleviate this inflammation is to follow a metabolism rest diet and give your digestive system a vacation (Olivia M. Farr, 2015).

Chapter 3: Recipes for Smoothies and Salads

If you want to lose weight and you have a particular period within which you want to achieve it, then here are some recipes that are going to be helpful.

Green Smoothie

Total Prep & Cooking Time: 2 minutes

Yields: 1 serving

Nutrition Facts: Calories: 144 | Carbs: 28.2g | Protein: 3.4g | Fat: 2.9g | Fiber: 4.8g

Ingredients:

- One cup each of
    o   Almond milk
    o   Raw spinach
- One-third of a cup of strawberries
- One orange, peeled

Method:

1. Add the peeled orange, strawberries, almond milk, and raw spinach in a blender and blend everything until you get a smooth paste. You can add extra water if required to achieve the desired thickness.

2. Pour out the smoothie into a glass and serve.

Strawberry Banana Smoothie

Total Prep & Cooking Time: 5 minutes

Yields: 2 servings

Nutrition Facts: Calories: 198| Carbs: 30.8g | Protein: 5.9g | Fat: 7.1g | Fiber: 4.8g

Ingredients:

- Half a cup each of
  - Milk
  - Greek yogurt
- One banana, frozen and quartered
- Two cups of fresh strawberries, halved

Method:

1. Add the milk, Greek yogurt, banana, and strawberries into a high-powered blender and blend until you get a smooth mixture.

2. Pour the smoothie equally into two separate glasses and serve.

Notes:

- *Don't add ice to the smoothie as it can make it watery very quickly. Using frozen bananas will keep your smoothie cold.*

- *As you're using bananas and strawberries, there is no need to add any artificial sweetener.*

Salmon Citrus Salad

Total Prep & Cooking Time: 20 minutes

Yields: 6 servings

Nutrition Facts: Calories: 336 | Carbs: 20g | Protein: 17g | Fat: 21g | Fiber: 5g

Ingredients:

- One pound of Citrus Salmon (slow-roasted)
- Half of an English cucumber, sliced
- One tomato (large), sliced into a quarter of an inch thick pieces
- One grapefruit, peeled and cut into segments
- Two oranges, peeled and cut into segments
- Three beets, roasted and quartered
- One avocado
- Boston lettuce leaves
- Two tablespoons of red wine vinegar
- Half of a red onion
- Flakey salt
- Aleppo pepper flakes

For the Citrus Shallot Vinaigrette,

- Five tablespoons of olive oil (extra-virgin)
- One clove of garlic, smashed
- Salt and pepper
- One and a half tablespoons of rice wine vinegar
- Two tablespoons of orange juice or fresh lemon juice

- One tablespoon of shallot, minced

Method:

For preparing the Citrus Shallot Vinaigrette:

1. Add the ingredients for the vinaigrette in a bowl and whisk them together.

2. Keep the mixture aside.

For assembling the salad,

1. Add the onions and vinegar in a small bowl and pickle them by letting them sit for about fifteen minutes.

2. In the meantime, place the lettuce leaves on the serving plate.

3. Dice the avocado in half and eliminate the pit. Then scoop the flesh and add them onto the plate. Sprinkle a dash of flakey salt and Aleppo pepper on top to season it.

4. Add the quartered beets onto the serving plate along with the grapefruit and orange segments.

5. Salt the cucumber and tomato slices lightly and add them onto the plate.

6. Then, scatter the pickled onions on top and cut the salmon into bits and add it on the plate.

7. Lastly, drizzle the Citrus Shallot Vinaigrette on top of the salad and finish off with a dash of flakey salt.

Chapter 4: Quick and Easy Breakfast and Main Course Recipes

Quinoa Salad

Total Prep & Cooking Time: 40 minutes

Yields: Eight servings

Nutrition Facts: Calories: 205 | Carbs: 25.9g | Protein: 6.1g | Fat: 9.4g | Fiber: 4.6g

Ingredients:

- One tablespoon of red wine vinegar
- One-fourth of a cup each of
  - Lemon juice (about two to three lemons)
  - Olive oil
- One cup each of
  - Quinoa (uncooked), rinsed with the help of a fine-mesh colander
  - Flat-leaf parsley (from a single large bunch), finely chopped
- Three-fourth of a cup of red onion (one small red onion), chopped
- One red bell pepper (medium-sized), chopped
- One cucumber (medium-sized), seeded and chopped
- One and a half cups of chickpeas (cooked), or One can of chickpeas (about fifteen ounces), rinsed and drained
- Two cloves of garlic, minced or pressed
- Two cups of water
- Black pepper, freshly ground
- Half a teaspoon of fine sea salt

Method:

1. Place a medium-sized saucepan over medium-high heat and add the rinsed quinoa into it along with the water. Allow the mixture to boil and then reduce the heat and simmer it. Cook for about fifteen minutes so that the quinoa has absorbed all the water. As time goes on, decrease the heat and maintain a gentle simmer. Take the saucepan away from the heat and cover it with a lid. Allow the cooked quinoa to rest for about five minutes to give it some time to increase in size.

2. Add the onions, bell pepper, cucumber, chickpeas, and parsley in a large serving bowl and mix them together. Keep the mixture aside.

3. Add the garlic, vinegar, lemon juice, olive oil, and salt in another small bowl and whisk the ingredients so that they are appropriately combined. Keep this mixture aside.

4. When the cooked quinoa has almost cooled down, transfer it to the serving bowl. Add the dressing on top and toss to combine everything together.

5. Add an extra pinch of sea salt and the black pepper to season according to your preference. Allow the salad to rest for five to ten minutes before serving it for the best results.

6. You can keep the salad in the refrigerator for up to four days. Make sure to cover it properly.

7. You can serve it at room temperature or chilled.

Notes: Instead of cooking additional quinoa, you can use about three cups of leftover quinoa for making this salad. Moreover, you can also serve this salad with fresh greens and an additional drizzle of lemon juice and olive oil. You can also add a dollop of cashew sour cream or crumbled feta cheese as a topping.

Herb and Goat Cheese Omelet

Total Prep & Cooking Time: 20 minutes

Yields: Two servings

Nutrition Facts: Calories: 233 | Carbs: 3.6g | Protein: 16g | Fat: 17.6g | Fiber: 1g

Ingredients:

- Half a cup each of
  - Red bell peppers (3 x quarter-inch), julienne-cut
  - Zucchini, thinly sliced
- Four large eggs
- Two teaspoons of olive oil, divided
- One-fourth of a cup of goat cheese (one ounce), crumbled
- Half a teaspoon of fresh tarragon, chopped
- One teaspoon each of
  - Fresh parsley, chopped
  - Fresh chives, chopped
- One-eighth of a teaspoon of salt
- One-fourth of a teaspoon of black pepper, freshly ground (divided)
- One tablespoon of water

Method:

1. Break the eggs into a bowl and add one tablespoon of water into it. Whisk them together and add in one-eighth of a teaspoon each of salt and ground black pepper.

2. In another small bowl, mix the goat cheese, tarragon, and parsley and keep it aside.

3. Place a nonstick skillet over medium heat and heat one teaspoon of olive oil in it. Add in the sliced zucchini, bell pepper, and the remaining one-eighth of a teaspoon of black pepper along with a dash of salt. Cook for about four minutes so that the bell pepper and zucchini get soft. Transfer the zucchini-bell pepper mixture onto a plate and cover it with a lid to keep it warm.

4. Add about half a teaspoon of oil into a skillet and add in half of the whisked egg into it. Do not stir the eggs and let the egg set slightly. Loosen the set edges of the omelet carefully with the help of a spatula. Tilt the skillet to move the uncooked part of the egg to the side. Keep following this method for about five seconds so that there is no more runny egg in the skillet. Add half of the crumbled goat cheese mixture evenly over the omelet and let it cook for another minute so that it sets.

5. Transfer the omelet onto a plate and fold it into thirds.

6. Repeat the process with the rest of the egg mixture, half a teaspoon of olive oil, and the goat cheese mixture.

7. Add the chopped chives on top of the omelets and serve with the bell pepper and zucchini mixture.

Mediterranean Cod

Total Prep & Cooking Time: 15 minutes

Yields: 4 servings

Nutrition Facts: Calories: 320 | Carbs: 31g | Protein: 35g | Fat: 8g | Fiber: 8g

Ingredients:

- One pound of spinach
- Four fillets of cod (almost one and a half pounds)
- Two zucchinis (medium-sized), chopped
- One cup of marinara sauce
- One-fourth of a teaspoon of red pepper, crushed
- Two cloves of garlic, chopped
- One tablespoon of olive oil
- Salt and pepper, according to taste
- Whole wheat roll, for serving

Method:

1. Place a ten-inch skillet on medium heat and add the marinara sauce and zucchini into it. Combine them together and let it simmer on medium heat.

2. Add the fillets of cod into the simmering sauce. Add one-fourth of a teaspoon each of salt and pepper too. Cover the skillet with a lid and let it cook for about seven minutes so that the cod gets just opaque throughout.

3. In the meantime, place a five-quart saucepot on medium heat and heat the olive oil in it. Add in the crushed red pepper and minced garlic. Stir and cook for about a minute.

4. Then, add in the spinach along with one-eighth of a teaspoon of salt. Cover the saucepot with a lid and let it cook for about five minutes, occasionally stirring so that the spinach gets wilted.

5. Add the spinach on the plates and top with the sauce and cod mixture and serve with the whole wheat roll.

Grilled Chicken and Veggies

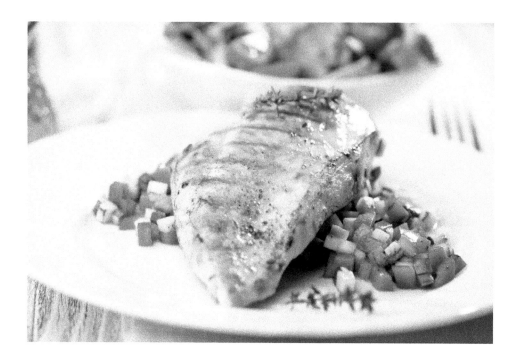

Total Prep & Cooking Time: 35 minutes

Yields: 4 servings

Nutrition Facts: Calories: 305 | Carbs: 11g | Protein: 26g | Fat: 17g | Fiber: 3g

Ingredients:

For the marinade,

- Four cloves of garlic, crushed

- One-fourth of a cup each of
  - Fresh lemon juice
  - Olive oil
- One teaspoon each of
  - Salt
  - Smoked paprika
  - Dried oregano
- Black pepper, according to taste
- Half a teaspoon of red chili flakes

For the grilling,

- Two to three zucchinis or courgette (large), cut into thin slices
- Twelve to sixteen spears of asparagus, woody sides trimmed
- Broccoli
- Two bell peppers, seeds eliminated and cut into thin slices
- Four pieces of chicken breasts (large), skinless and de-boned

Method:

1. Preheat your griddle or grill pan.

2. Sprinkle some salt on top of the chicken breasts to season them. Keep them aside to rest while you prepare the marinade.

3. For the marinade, mix all the ingredients properly.

4. Add about half of the marinade over the vegetables and the other half over the seasoned chicken breasts. Allow the marinade to rest for a couple of minutes.

5. Place the chicken pieces on the preheated grill. Grill for about five to seven minutes on each side until they are cooked according to your preference. The time on the grill depends on the thickness of the chicken breasts.

6. Remove them from the grill and cover them using a foil. Set it aside to rest and prepare to grill the vegetables in the meantime.

7. Grill the vegetables for a few minutes until they begin to char and are crispy yet tender.

8. Remove them from the grill and transfer them onto a serving plate. Serve the veggies along with the grilled chicken and add the lemon wedges on the side for squeezing.

Notes: You can add as much or as little vegetables as you like. The vegetable amounts are given only as a guide. Moreover, feel free to replace some of them with the vegetables you like to eat.

Stuffed Peppers

Total Prep & Cooking Time: 50 minutes

Yields: 4 servings

Nutrition Facts: Calories: 438 | Carbs: 32g | Protein: 32g | Fat: 20g | Fiber: 5g

Ingredients:

For the stuffed peppers,

- One pound of ground chicken or turkey
- Four bell peppers (large) of any color
- One and a quarter of a cups of cheese, shredded
- One and a half cups of brown rice, cooked (you can use cauliflower rice or quinoa)
- One can (about fourteen ounces) of fire-roasted diced tomatoes along with its juices
- Two teaspoons of olive oil (extra-virgin)
- One teaspoon each of
  - Garlic powder
  - Ground cumin
- One tablespoon of ground chili powder
- One-fourth of a teaspoon of black pepper
- Half a teaspoon of kosher salt

For serving,

- Sour cream or Greek yogurt
- Salsa
- Freshly chopped cilantro
- Avocado, sliced
- Freshly squeezed lemon juice

Method:

1. Preheat your oven to 375 degrees Fahrenheit.

2. Take a nine by thirteen-inch baking dish and coat it lightly with a nonstick cooking spray.

3. Take the bell peppers and slice them from top to bottom into halves. Remove the membranes and the seeds. Keep the bell peppers in the baking dish with the cut-side facing upwards.

4. Place a large, nonstick skillet on medium-high heat and heat the olive oil in it. Add in the chicken, pepper, salt, garlic powder, ground cumin, and chili powder and cook for about four minutes so that the chicken is cooked through and gets brown. Break apart the chicken while it's cooking. Drain off any excess liquid and then add in the can of diced tomatoes along with the juices. Allow it to simmer for a minute.

5. Take the pan away from the heat. Add in the cooked rice along with three-fourth of a cup of the shredded cheese and stir everything together.

6. Add this filling inside the peppers and add the remaining shredded cheese as a topping.

7. Add a little amount of water into the pan containing the peppers so that it barely covers the bottom of the pan.

8. Keep it uncovered and bake it in the oven for twenty-five to thirty-five minutes so that the cheese gets melted and the peppers get soft.

9. Add any of your favorite fixings as a topping and serve hot.

Notes:

- *For preparing the stuffed peppers ahead of time, make sure to allow the rice and chicken mixture to cool down completely before filling the peppers. You can prepare the stuffed peppers before time, and then you have to cover it with a lid and keep it in the refrigerator for a maximum of twenty-four hours before baking the peppers.*

- *If you're planning to reheat the stuffed peppers, gently reheat them in your oven or microwave. If you're using a microwave for this purpose, make sure to cut the peppers into pieces to warm them evenly.*

- *You can store any leftovers in the freezer for up to three months. Alternatively, you can keep them in the refrigerator for up to four days. Allow it to thaw in the fridge overnight.*

Brussels Sprouts With Honey Mustard Chicken

Total Prep & Cooking Time: Fifty minutes

Yields: Four servings

Nutrition Facts: Calories: 360 | Carbs: 14.5g | Protein: 30.8g | Fat: 20g | Fiber: 3.7g

Ingredients:

- One and a half pounds of Brussels sprouts, divided into two halves
- Two pounds of chicken thighs, skin-on and bone-in (about four medium-sized thighs)
- Three cloves of garlic, minced
- One-fourth of a large onion, cut into slices
- One tablespoon each of
    o Honey
    o Whole-grain mustard
    o Dijon mustard
- Two tablespoons of freshly squeezed lemon juice (one lemon)
- One-fourth of a cup plus two tablespoons of olive oil (extra-virgin)
- Freshly ground black pepper
- Kosher salt
- Non-stick cooking spray

Method:

1. Preheat your oven to 425 degrees Fahrenheit.

2. Take a large baking sheet and grease it with nonstick cooking spray. Keep it aside.

3. Add the minced garlic, honey, whole-grain mustard, Dijon mustard, one tablespoon of the lemon juice, one-fourth cup of the olive oil in a medium-sized bowl and mix them together. Add the Kosher salt and black pepper to season according to your preference.

4. Dip the chicken thighs into the sauce with the help of tongs and coat both sides. Transfer the things on the baking sheet. You can get rid of any extra sauce.

5. Mix the red onion and Brussels sprouts in a medium-sized bowl and drizzle one tablespoon of lemon juice along with the remaining two tablespoons of olive oil onto it. Toss everything together until the vegetables are adequately coated.

6. Place the red onion-Brussels sprouts mixture on the baking sheet around the chicken pieces. Ensure that the chicken and vegetables are not overlapping.

7. Sprinkle a little amount of salt and pepper on the top and keep it in the oven to roast for about thirty to thirty-five minutes so that the Brussels sprouts get crispy and the chicken has an internal temperature of 165 degrees Fahrenheit and has turned golden brown.

8. Serve hot.

Quinoa Stuffed Chicken

Total Prep & Cooking Time: 50 minutes

Yields: Four servings

Nutrition Facts: Calories: 355 | Carbs: 28g | Protein: 30g | Fat: 13g | Fiber: 4g

Ingredients:

- One and a half cups of chicken broth
- Three-fourths of a cup of quinoa (any color of your choice)
- Four chicken breasts (boneless and skinless)
- One lime, zested and one tablespoon of lime juice
- One-fourth of a cup of cilantro, chipped
- One-third of a cup of unsweetened coconut, shaved or coconut chips
- One Serrano pepper, seeded and diced
- Two cloves of garlic, minced
- Half a cup of red onion, diced
- Three-fourth of a cup of bell pepper, diced
- One tablespoon of coconut oil
- One teaspoon each of
  - Salt
  - Chili powder
  - Ground cumin

Method:

1. Preheat your oven to 375 degrees Fahrenheit.

2. Take a rimmed baking sheet and line it with parchment paper.

3. Place a medium-sized saucepan over medium-high heat and add the coconut oil in it. After it has melted, add in the Serrano peppers, garlic, red onion, and bell pepper and sauté for about one to two minutes so that they soften just a bit. Make sure that the vegetables are still bright in color. Then transfer the cooked vegetables into a bowl.

4. Add the quinoa in the empty sauce pot and increase the heat to high. Pour the chicken broth in it along with half a teaspoon of salt. Close the lid of the pot and bring it to a boil, allowing the quinoa to cook for about fifteen minutes so that the surface of the quinoa develops vent holes, and the broth has absorbed completely. Take the pot away from the heat and allow it to steam for an additional five minutes.

5. In the meantime, cut a slit along the long side in each chicken breast. It will be easier with the help of a boning knife. You are making a deep pocket in each breast, having a half-inch border around the remaining three attached sides. Keep the knife parallel to the cutting board and cut through the middle of the breast and leaving the opposite side attached. Try to cut it evenly as it's challenging to cook thick uncut portions properly in the oven. After that, add salt, cumin, and chili powder on all sides of the chicken.

6. When the quinoa has turned fluffy, add in the lime juice, lime zest, shaved coconut, and sautéed vegetables and stir them in. Taste the mixture and adjust the salt as per your preference.

7. Add the confetti quinoa mixture inside the cavity of the chicken breast. Place the stuffed breasts on the baking sheet with the quinoa facing upwards. They'll look like open envelopes.

8. Bake them in the oven for about twenty minutes.

9. Serve warm.

Kale and Sweet Potato Frittata

Total Prep & Cooking Time: 30 minutes

Yields: 4 servings

Nutrition Facts: Calories: 144 | Carbs: 10g | Protein: 7g | Fat: 9g | Fiber: 2g

Ingredients:

- Three ounces of goat cheese
- Two cloves of garlic
- Half of a red onion (small)
- Two cups each of
  - Sweet potatoes
  - Firmly packed kale, chopped
- Two tablespoons of olive oil
- One cup of half-and-half
- Six large eggs
- Half a teaspoon of pepper, freshly ground
- One teaspoon of Kosher salt

Method:

1. Preheat your oven to 350 degrees Fahrenheit.

2. Add the eggs, half-and-half, salt, and black pepper in a bowl and whisk everything together.

3. Place a ten-inch ovenproof nonstick skillet over medium heat and add one tablespoon of oil in it. Sauté the sweet potatoes in the skillet for about eight to ten minutes so that they turn soft and golden brown. Transfer them onto a plate and keep warm.

4. Next, add in the remaining one tablespoon of oil and sauté the kale along with the red onions and garlic in it for about three to four minutes so that the kale gets soft and wilted. Then, add in the whisked egg mixture evenly over the vegetables and cook for an additional three minutes.

5. Add some goat cheese on the top and bake it in the oven for ten to fourteen minutes so that it sets.

Walnut, Ginger, and Pineapple Oatmeal

Total Prep & Cooking Time: 30 minutes

Yields: 4 servings

Nutrition Facts: Calories: 323 | Carbs: 61g | Protein: 6g | Fat: 8g | Fiber: 5g

Ingredients:

- Two large eggs
- Two cups each of
  - Fresh pineapple, coarsely chopped
  - Old-fashioned rolled oats
  - Whole milk
- One cup of walnuts, chopped
- Half a cup of maple syrup
- One piece of ginger
- Two teaspoons of vanilla extract
- Half a teaspoon of salt

Method:

1. Preheat your oven to 400 degrees Fahrenheit.

2. Add the ginger, walnuts, pineapple, oats, and salt in a large bowl and mix them together. Add the mixture evenly among four ten-ounce ramekins and keep them aside.

3. Whisk the eggs along with the milk, maple syrup, and vanilla extract in a medium-sized bowl. Pour one-quarter of this mixture into each ramekin containing the oat-pineapple mixture.

4. Keep the ramekins on the baking sheet and bake them in the oven for about twenty-five minutes until the oats turn light golden brown on the top and have set properly.

5. Serve with some additional maple syrup on the side.

Caprese Salad

Total Prep & Cooking Time: 15 minutes

Yields: 4 servings

Nutrition Facts: Calories: 216 | Carbs: 4g | Protein: 13g | Fat: 16g | Fiber: 1g

Ingredients:

For the salad,

- Nine basil leaves (medium-sized)
- Eight ounces of fresh whole-milk mozzarella cheese
- Two tomatoes (medium-sized)
- One-fourth of a teaspoon of black pepper, freshly ground
- Half a teaspoon of Kosher salt, or one-fourth of a teaspoon of sea salt

For the dressing,

- One teaspoon of Dijon mustard
- One tablespoon each of
  - Balsamic vinegar
  - Olive oil

Method:

1. Add the olive oil, balsamic vinegar, and Dijon mustard into a small bowl and whisk them together with the help of a small hand whisk so that you get a smooth salad dressing. Keep it aside.

2. Cut the tomatoes into thin slices and try to get ten slices in total.

3. Cut the mozzarella into nine thin slices with the help of a sharp knife.

4. Place the slices of tomatoes and mozzarella on a serving plate, alternating and overlapping one another. Then, add the basil leaves on the top.

5. Season the salad with black pepper and salt and drizzle the prepared dressing on top.

6. Serve immediately.

One-Pot Chicken Soup

Total Prep & Cooking Time: 30 minutes

Yields: 6 servings

Nutrition Facts: Calories: 201 | Carbs: 20g | Protein: 16g | Fat: 7g | Fiber: 16g

Ingredients:

- Three cups of loosely packed chopped kale (or other greens of your choice)
- Two cups of chicken, shredded
- One can of white beans (about fifteen ounces), slightly drained
- Eight cups of broth (vegetable broth or chicken broth)
- Four cloves of garlic, minced
- One cup of yellow or white onion, diced
- One tablespoon of avocado oil (skip if you are using bacon)
- One strip of uncured bacon, chopped (optional)
- Black pepper + sea salt, according to taste

Method:

1. Place a Dutch oven or a large pot over medium heat. When it gets hot, add in the oil or bacon (optional), stirring occasionally, and allow it to get hot for about a minute.

2. Then, add in the diced onion and sauté for four to five minutes, occasionally stirring so that the onions get fragrant and translucent. Add in the minced garlic next and sauté for another two to three minutes. Be careful so as not to burn the ingredients.

3. Then, add the chicken, slightly drained white beans, and broth and bring the mixture to a simmer. Cook for about ten minutes to bring out all the flavors. Taste the mixture and add salt and pepper to season according to your preference. Add in the chopped kale in the last few minutes of cooking. Cover the pot and let it cook until the kale has wilted.

4. Serve hot.

Notes: You can store any leftovers in the freezer for up to a month. Or, you can store them in the refrigerator for a maximum of three to four days. Simply reheat on the stovetop or in the microwave and eat it later.

Chocolate Pomegranate Truffles

Total Prep & Cooking Time: 10 minutes

Yields: Twelve to Fourteen truffles

Nutrition Facts: Calories: 95 | Carbs: 26g | Protein: 1g | Fat: 2g | Fiber: 3g

Ingredients:

- One-third of a cup of pomegranate arils
- Half a teaspoon each of
  - Vanilla extract
  - Ground cinnamon
- Half a cup of ground flax seed
- Two tablespoons of cocoa powder (unsweetened)
- About one tablespoon of water
- One and a half cups of pitted Medjool dates
- One-eighth of a teaspoon of salt

Method:

1. Add the pitted dates in a food processor and blend until it begins to form a ball. Add some water and pulse again. Add in the vanilla, cinnamon, flax seeds, cocoa powder, and salt and blend until everything is combined properly.

2. Turn off the food processor and unplug it. Add in the pomegranate arils and fold them in the mixture so that they are distributed evenly.

3. Make twelve to fourteen balls using the mixture. You can create an outer coating or topping if you want by rolling the balls in finely shredded coconut or cocoa powder.

Notes: *You can store the chocolate pomegranate truffles in the fridge in an air-tight container for a maximum of three days.*

PART III

This chapter will give you a brief introduction to what the Hashimoto disease is and what diet you can follow in this case.

Chapter 1: Causes and Symptoms of Hashimoto Disease

Hashimoto's disease is a type of autoimmune disorder. It may lead to hypothyroidism (i.e., underactive thyroid). When you have this disease, your thyroid gets attacked by your immune system. It causes immense damage to the thyroid gland as a result of which it fails to produce an adequate amount of thyroid hormones. Hashimoto's disease causes inflammation (chronic lymphocytic thyroiditis), which eventually leads to hypothyroidism. Men and women of all ages and even children can get affected by this disease. Middle-aged women are more likely to get affected by this particular disease. Generally, a thyroid function test is suggested by the doctors for the detection of Hashimoto's disease. This disease can be treated by a simple thyroid hormone replacement effectively.

A study stated that earlier, it was a little difficult for the doctors to detect Hashimoto's disease. But now it can be easily identified by an antibody test (since this disease causes the production of harmful antibodies) and a hormone test (during hypothyroidism, the thyroid hormone level is low, whereas the level of TSH is more). The pituitary glands release more TSH so that it can stimulate the thyroid to increase the production of the thyroid hormone.

- People who get exposed to enormous amounts of radiation are more likely to develop Hashimoto's disease.

- Having an underlying medical condition often acts as a triggering factor in the case of developing new health issues. If you already have an autoimmune disease like type-1 diabetes or rheumatoid arthritis, then you are more prone to Hashimoto's disease.

- Heredity is an important factor when it comes to autoimmune diseases. So, if there is Hashimoto's disease in your family history, then you have a fair chance of developing the same.

- People of all ages can get affected by Hashimoto's disease, but middle-aged people are at higher risk.

- Gender is also a factor as women are more prone to this particular disease.

Symptoms of Hashimoto's Disease

Hashimoto's disease can be asymptomatic at the beginning, but it slowly starts showing you symptoms after a few days. Let's see some of the symptoms of this disease.

- Memory lapse

- Depression

- Heavy menstrual bleeding (can also be prolonged)

- Muscle fatigue

- Pain in the joints and stiffness

- Muscle aches, stiffness, and tenderness

- Uncontrollable weight gain

- Tongue enlargement

- Loss of hair

- Nails become brittle

- The face becomes puffed up

- Dry and pale skin

- Constipation

- Hypersensitivity to cold

- Sluggishness and fatigue

Supplements That You Can Take

Millions of individuals are surviving in this world who is suffering from Hashimoto's Disease or Hashimoto thyroiditis. This deep-rooted autoimmune situation makes the thyroid gland inactive. It is true that Hashimoto Disease develops or progresses slowly. But, such autoimmune condition attacks as well as destroys the thyroid gland. The symptoms of this disease might remain unnoticed for many years. Treatment begins after checking levels of one-two antibodies, namely thyroglobulin (Tg) and thyroperoxidase (TPO). In certain cases, the thyroid gland might also be checked through ultrasound. But, you need not worry as you may survive well even with this disease. Besides medical intervention, various supplements are available that play a crucial role in dealing with Hashimoto Disease.

But, before consuming any such supplements, it is better to consult your healthcare provider or practitioner. He or she is the perfect person who will be able to guide you according to your health condition. Here you will get to know about some of the essential supplements that you may consume for Hashimoto Disease.

- **Selenium**- Selenium assists the thyroid gland in producing thyroid hormone. It is also helpful in converting T4 (thyroxine) into T3 (triiodothyronine). Various studies have revealed the fact that selenium supplementation is effective for treating this disease, whether combined with levothyroxine or used alone. Selenium supplements are beneficial, but it is better not to consume more than one hundred micrograms (mcg) each day. You may intake more or less than the mentioned quantity only if your doctor prescribes you to do so. For more trust-worthy selenium consumption, it is better to rely on supplements than food sources.

- **Zinc**- In accordance with certain reliable research, supplementation of zinc might help maintain a healthy thyroid hormone level. Expert healthcare providers usually suggest fifteen to thirty mg of zinc supplement daily. Zinc and selenium together are worthy of improving the functioning of the thyroid.

- **Omega-3 Fatty Acid**- It is believed that omega-3 fatty acids, particularly docosahexaenoic acid (DHA) and icosapentaenoic acid (EPA) are helpful for individual suffering from autoimmune thyroid conditions. It is recommended to consume fish oil supplements twice or thrice a week. Omega-3 fatty acid supplement (plant-based) is also beneficial but is not so well absorbed like fish oil supplements.

- **Vitamin B1**- Evidence exists that thiamine or vitamin B1 supplements are useful in reducing fatigue of those people having Hashimoto's thyroiditis. This disease leads to decreased thiamine absorption. If you are facing such a problem, you may discuss it with your physician for the dosage of thiamine supplementation.

Chapter 2: Recipes for Appetizers and Snacks

Oven Roasted Okra

Total Prep & Cooking Time: 35 minutes

Yields: Four servings

Nutrition Facts: Calories: 104 | Carbs: 9.4g | Protein: 2.2g | Fat: 7.2g | Fiber: 3.6g

Ingredients:

- One pound of okra
- One tbsp. each of
  - Lemon juice
  - Balsamic vinegar
- One teaspoon each of
  - Onion powder
  - Garlic powder
- A quarter teaspoon of black pepper
- Two tablespoons of avocado oil
- A three-fourth teaspoon of sea salt

Method:

1. Set the oven temperature at 400 degrees F. You will require a baking sheet to bake the okra. With a parchment paper, line the sheet.

2. Rinse the okras thoroughly under running water and dry them. Chop off the head of each okra. Slice each okra into five pieces and then set them aside.

3. Place the okra pieces evenly on the sheet and top them with salt, pepper, lemon, oil, and balsamic vinegar. Toss them well so that the okra is entirely coated with the seasonings.

4. Transfer the sheet to an oven and roast them for twenty-four to twenty-five minutes. Flip the pieces in between to cook both sides evenly.

5. Take the sheet off the oven and then allow them to cool down.

6. Serve and enjoy.

Note: *Okra is an incredibly delicious summer vegetable.*

Honeydew Smoothie Bowl

Total Prep & Cooking Time: 5 minutes

Yields: 2 servings

Nutrition Facts: Calories: 176 | Carbs: 41.4g | Protein: 2.5g | Fat: 1.6g | Fiber: 3g

Ingredients:

- One tbsp. of honey
- One-third cup of green juice of your choice (for example, wheatgrass)
- Half a cup of coconut milk beverage (unsweetened)
- Four cups of cubed honeydew (frozen, make pieces of half an inch in size)
- Salt as per taste
- For garnishing – nuts, fresh basil, berries, and melon balls

Method:

1. Use a high-speed blender or food processor to blend the following ingredients together – salt, honey, juice, coconut milk, and honeydew. Stop in between blending and pulsing to scrape down the sides of the food processor.

2. Pulse for about one to two minutes to get your desired consistency. Before serving, top the smoothie with toppings of your choice.

Wake-Up Smoothie

Total Prep & Cooking Time: 5 minutes

Yields: 3 servings

Nutrition Facts: Calories: 139 | Carbs: 28g | Protein: 4.4g | Fat: 2g | Fiber: 4.3g

Ingredients:

- One banana
- 1.25 cups of orange juice (if possible, then calcium-fortified)
- Half a cup of silken tofu (low-fat) or low-fat yogurt
- 1.25 cups of frozen berries such as blackberries, raspberries, strawberries, or blueberries
- One tbsp. of sugar or Stevia

Method:

1. In the bowl of a blender, add the ingredients.
2. Cover the bowl and blend the ingredients until you get a smooth and creamy mixture.
3. Serve and enjoy!

Cucumber Radish Salsa

Total Prep Time: 10 minutes

Yields: Four plates of salsa

Nutrition Facts: Calories: 22 | Carb: 4.7g | Protein: 0.9g | Fat: 0.4g | Fiber: 1.6g

Ingredients:

- One large-sized cucumber (sliced)
- A quarter cup of chopped cilantro
- Two juiced limes
- One heaping cup of radishes, eight to ten regular (either sliced into thin halves or diced)
- Three tablespoons of diced red onion
- One tablespoon of olive oil
- To taste: Pepper (freshly ground and optional) and salt

Method:

1. In a bowl, place all the veggies listed in the ingredients section.

2. Combine them thoroughly, and place them in a refrigerator for one hour before serving.

Crispy Oven-Fried Fish Tacos

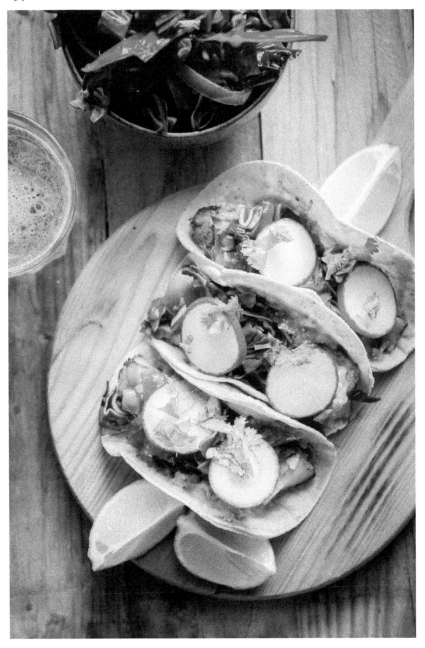

Total Prep & Cooking Time: 45 minutes

Yields: 4 servings (Two tacos per serving)

Nutrition Facts: Calories: 496 | Carbs: 65.4g | Protein: 27.3g | Fat: 17.6g | Fiber: 15.2g

Ingredients:

- A cup of cereal flakes (whole-grain)
- Cooking spray
- Half a tsp. each of
  - Salt (keep it divided)
  - Paprika
  - Garlic powder
- Half a cup of all-purpose flour
- Three-quarter tsp. of freshly ground pepper (keep it divided)
- Three-quarter cups of breadcrumbs (whole wheat)
- Two egg whites
- One lb. of cod (cut into strips)
- Two tbsps. each of
  - Avocado oil
  - Water
  - Unseasoned rice vinegar
- One avocado (sliced)
- Pico de gallo
- Three cups of coleslaw mix
- Eight warmed corn tortillas

Method:

1. Set the temperature of the oven to 450 degrees F and preheat. Take a baking sheet and, on it, place a wire rack. Use cooking spray to coat it nicely.

2. In the bowl of a food processor, add the breadcrumbs, cereal flakes, paprika, garlic powder, half a tsp. of pepper, and half a tsp. of salt. Process all these ingredients until you get a smooth mixture. Take this mixture and spread it on a shallow dish.

3. Take another shallow dish and place flour on it. Then, in the third shallow dish, whisk water and egg together.

4. Take each fillet of fish, dredge it in flour, and then dip the fillet in the egg mixture. Then, coat both sides of the fillets with breadcrumbs evenly.

5. Once done, place these fillets on the greased wire racks. The breaded fish should be coated with cooking spray as well. Bake them for about ten minutes by the end of which they should become golden brown and crispy.

6. Meanwhile, take a medium-sized bowl and, in it, whisk the following ingredients together – remaining pepper and salt, vinegar, and oil. Add the mix of coleslaw to it and toss nicely so that everything is evenly coated.

7. Finally, take the tortillas, divide the avocados, coleslaw mix, and fish evenly. If you want, then serve them with pico de gallo.

Strawberry Mango Salsa

Total Prep Time: 10 minutes

Yields: Four servings

Nutrition Facts: Calories: 126 | Carbs: 20.3g | Protein: 1.8g | Fat: 5.7g | Fiber: 4.6g

Ingredients:

- One cup of diced strawberries
- A quarter cup of diced red onions
- A tablespoon of chopped cilantro
- One medium-sized mango (chopped)
- One medium avocado (sliced)
- One lime, juiced
- To taste: Salt

Method:

1. In a bowl (medium-sized), add all ingredients listed in the section, except the salt. Carefully combine them with spatula's help so that the veggies get well coated with the lime juice. Make sure that you do not crush the avocado pieces.

2. After the ingredients have been entirely tossed, sprinkle over the salt. You can serve immediately, or you can store in the refrigerator in a closed container.

Strawberry Mousse

Total Prep & Cooking Time: 6 hours and 30 minutes

Yields: Six servings

Nutrition Facts: Calories: 100 | Carbs: 20g | Protein: 5g | Fat: 0g | Fiber: 1g

Ingredients:

- Twelve ounces of halved and hulled fresh strawberries
- A three-fourth cup of Greek yogurt
- Lemon juice (few drops)
- One-third cup of honey
- Four egg whites
- Salt to taste

Method:

1. Place strawberries and honey in a blender and make them smooth. Put them in a bowl.

2. Pour the yogurt in the bowl and whisk them properly.

3. Take another bowl. Add the lemon splash, salt, and egg whites. Using a hand mixer, whisk the eggs to form stiff peaks such a way that the egg remains intact when turned upside down.

4. With a spatula, mix one-third of the egg mixture with strawberry. Slowly pour the rest of the egg whites mixture, ensuring that the bubbles do not break.

5. Transfer to six containers. Store the containers for six hours in the refrigerator. Enjoy.

Grilled Salmon and Veggies

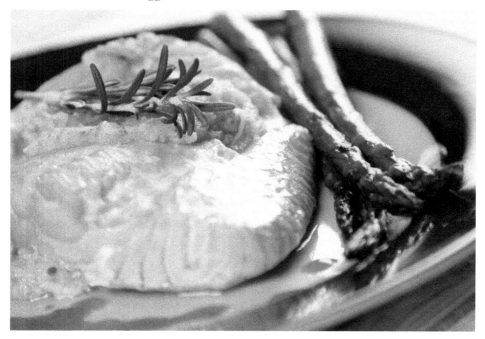

Total Prep & Cooking Time: 25 minutes

Yields: Four servings

Nutrition Facts: Calories: 281 | Carbs: 10.6g | Protein: 30.2g | Fat: 2.3g | Fiber: 3.1g

Ingredients:

- One medium-sized zucchini, sliced vertically into halves
- One onion (cut into wedges of one-inch), red

- Half a tsp. of salt
- One and a quarter lb. of salmon fillets (sliced into portions of four)
- One lemon, sliced into wedges of four
- Two bell peppers (each of red, orange, yellow), halved, seeded, and trimmed
- One tbsp. of olive oil (extra-virgin)
- Half a tsp. of pepper (ground)
- A quarter cup of fresh basil (thinly sliced)

Method:

1. Keep the grill preheated to moderate heat.

2. Place onions, pepper, and zucchini in a bowl sprinkle some salt (a quarter tsp.) and brush them with oil.

3. Place the salmon fillets in another bowl and sprinkle with remaining salt and pepper.

4. Transfer the salmon and the veggies to grill and then cook the vegetables occasionally, turning and cooking each side for six minutes until they tenderize. Cook the salmon for ten minutes until they flake.

5. Remove the vegetables and chop them into small pieces when they have cooled down. Toss them well. Serve the salmon aside the vegetables. Garnish them with one tbsp. of basil and the lemon wedges.

Chapter 3: Main Course Recipes

Zucchini Noodles With Shrimp and Avocado Pesto

Total Prep & Cooking Time: 35 minutes

Yields: 4 servings (1.75 cups each serving)

Nutrition Facts: Calories: 446 | Carbs: 15.8g | Protein: 25.9g | Fat: 33.2g | Fiber: 6.6g

Ingredients:

- One avocado (ripe)
- One cup of basil leaves (fresh)
- Three-quarter tsp. of salt (keep it divided)
- Five-six zucchini (medium-sized, trimmed)
- A quarter cup of pistachios (shelled, unsalted)
- Three garlic cloves (minced)
- A quarter cup of olive oil (extra-virgin variety, + two tbsps. extra)
- A quarter tsp. of freshly ground pepper
- 1-2 tsps. of Old Bay seasoning
- One lb. of raw shrimp (deveined and peeled)
- Two tbsps. of lemon juice

Method:

1. Your first step is to prepare the zucchini using a spiralizer and form thin strips. Then, take the zoodles and place them in a colander. Sprinkle half a tsp. of salt. Allow it to drain for half an hour and squeeze to remove any excess water.

2. In a food processor, combine the following – pepper, lemon juice, pistachios basil, avocado, and a quarter tsp. of salt. Make sure everything is finely chopped. To make it smooth, add a quarter cup of oil.

3. In a large-sized skillet, heat one tbsp. of oil on medium-high flame. Cook the garlic in the heated oil for about thirty seconds. Then, sprinkle the Old Bay seasoning and add the shrimp. Keep stirring and cook the shrimp for about four minutes. Once done, transfer the shrimp to a bowl.

4. Take the remaining one tbsp. of oil and add it to the pan. The zoodles should have drained by now, so you have to add them to the pan and toss them for about three minutes. Then, transfer them to the bowl containing shrimp and mix properly. Add the pesto and combine it by tossing everything once again. Serve and enjoy!

Honey Ginger Shrimp Bowls

Total Prep & cooking Time: 26 minutes

Yields: Two bowls

Nutrition Facts: Calories: 165.9 | Carbs: 4.1g | Protein: 19g | Fat: 8.1g | Fiber: 0.8g

Ingredients:

For preparing the shrimp,

- Twelve ounces of large deveined and peeled shrimp (uncooked)
- One teaspoon of freshly minced ginger
- Two teaspoons of avocado oil
- Two tablespoons each of
  - Honey
  - Coconut aminos
- Two cloves of garlic (diced)
- To taste: salt, lime, pepper (ground freshly, optional)

Dressing ingredients,

- Two tablespoons each of
  - Olive oil
  - Lime juice
- A quarter teaspoon each of

- o Ginger powder
- o Garlic powder
- One teaspoon each of
  - o Coconut aminos
  - o Honey
- To taste – Pepper and salt

Salad ingredients,

- Four cups of spinach or arugula
- Four onions sliced (green)
- One avocado (diced)
- Half a cup each of
  - o Carrots (shredded)
  - o Radishes (shredded)
- A quarter of cilantro (sliced)

Method:

1. Take a bowl and put coconut aminos, ginger, honey, and garlic. Combine them well with a whisk.

2. Take a lidded container and pour the shrimp into it along with the marinade. Stir thoroughly.

3. Marinate the shrimp for two hours in the refrigerator.

4. After the period described above, pour some avocado oil in the skillet and heat over moderate flame. Pour the shrimp mixture into the skillet. Cook for about three minutes to make the shrimp opaque and then flip.

5. Continue cooking for an additional three minutes to make the sauce thickened—season with lime, pepper, and salt. Cook well to form an even coating over the shrimp pieces.

6. Toss carrots, greens, and radishes in a bowl and then divide equally into two plates.

7. To serve: top each dish with the cooked shrimp, cilantro, avocado, dressing, onions, and wedges.

Note: You can chop the carrots and radishes with shredding attachment or the box grater. Be careful while cooking the shrimp. The inner flesh must be white, and the outer tissue should turn pink.

Beef and Sweet Potatoes Stew

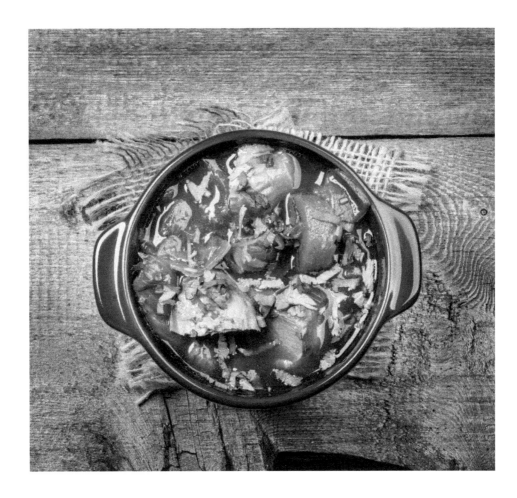

Total Prep & Cooking Time: 20 minutes

Yields: Four servings

Nutrition Facts: Calories: 195 | Carbs: 18g | Protein: 19g | Fat: 5g | Fiber: 3g

Ingredients:

- One teaspoon each of
  - Avocado oil
  - Salt
- One tablespoon of minced ginger
- Two teaspoons each of
  - Oregano (dried)
  - Thyme (dried)
- One cup each of
  - Pumpkin puree
  - Cilantro (chopped)
  - Carrots (sliced)
- One pound of grass-fed beef (ground)
- Diced avocado
- One diced onion
- Three cloves of garlic (minced)
- Five cups of cubed and peeled sweet potato
- Two cups bone broth
- Two limes juiced
- Six sliced green onions
- Pepper to taste and optional

Method:

1. Pour avocado oil in an instant pot and set the function to 'saute.' After oil starts to boil, add the ginger, carrots, onion, garlic, sweet potatoes, thyme, pepper, salt, and oregano, stir for few minutes until you get the smell.

2. Turn it off. Add the bone broth and the pumpkin puree to the mixture and beef (ground) to form a single layer at the bottom.

3. Cook the stew using the manual setting for five minutes. Release the method by switching to the quick-release mode.

4. Season with lime juice. Divide equally among four bowls and top with avocado and herbs to serve.

Roasted Sunchoke Salad

Total Prep & Cooking Time: 35 minutes

Yields: Four servings

Nutrition Facts: Calories: 143 | Carbs: 20g | Protein: 2g | Fat: 6g | Fiber: 2g

Ingredients:

- Two pounds of trimmed and scrubbed sunchokes
- Half a cup of minced red onion
- Two tablespoons of avocado oil
- A three-fourth cup of parsley (minced)
- One clove of garlic (diced)
- To taste: Black pepper (ground) and salt

Method:

1. Set the oven at a temperature of 425 degrees F. place a baking sheet on your countertop. Mix the sunchokes, pepper, salt, and one tbsp. of avocado oil. Toss them well over the baking sheet in an even layer.

2. Bake for thirty minutes, occasionally stirring until the edges turn brown and crispy, leaving the middle portions creamy.

3. Meanwhile, in a bowl, place the remaining ingredients and then add the sunchokes mixture. Stir them well and add some seasoning if required.

4. Serve immediately.

Kale Salad

Total Prep Time: 20 minutes

Yields: Four bowls of salad

Nutrition Facts: Calories: 334 | Carbs: 19g | Protein: 9g | Fat: 26g | Fiber: 4g

Ingredients:

- Five cups of chopped kale
- One-eighth tsp. of salt
- Half a cup each of
    o Cheese
    o Sliced almonds
- A quarter cup each of
    o Seeds of sunflower
    o Cranberries
    o Diced red onions
- Two tsps. of olive oil
- Two cups of chopped broccoli
- A quarter to a half cup of shredded carrots

For the lemon dressing,

- A quarter cup of oil (olive)
- One tbsp. of Dijon mustard
- Half a tsp. of oregano (dried)

- One-eighth tsp. of black pepper (ground)
- Two tbsps. each of
  - Lemon juice
  - Vinegar (red wine)
- One garlic clove (minced)
- A quarter tsp. of salt
- One tsp. of sugar or honey

Method:

1. Massage the chopped kale leaves with salt and oil. Brush them with the fingers to make the leaves become tender and darken in color.

2. For the dressing, mix all ingredients in the jar with a lid. Shake them well so that they emulsify. Adjust the sweetener, pepper, and salt as your heart desires.

3. Take a bowl and place broccoli, massaged kale, cheese, onion, almond, carrots, cranberries, and sunflower seeds. Toss them well. Pour the dressing ingredients over it (about one-third). Shake well to coat and then add the extra dressing according to your taste.

Taco Spaghetti Squash Boats

Total Prep & Cooking Time: 45 minutes

Yields: Four servings

Nutrition Facts: Calories: 553 | Carbs: 28g | Protein: 29.6g | Fat: 38.5g | Fiber: 9g

Ingredients:

- Two tbsps. of canola oil
- One cup each of
  o Onion (chopped)
  o Blended and shredded cheese (Mexican)
  o Chopped lettuce (romaine)
- One medium-sized tomato (diced)
- Two tsps. of cumin (ground)
- A quarter cup of prepared salsa (some extra for serving)
- One chopped avocado
- Three lb. of spaghetti squash, seeded and vertically sliced into halves
- Half a tsp. of salt
- Four tsps. of chili powder
- Three garlic (diced)
- One lb. of turkey (ground)

Method:

1. Set the oven at a temperature of 450 degrees F. Place a skillet over moderate flame and pour few oil drops. Then add the garlic, onion, and turkey. Cook for seven minutes, stirring occasionally and breaking the turkey chunks. Then add chili powder, salt, tomato, and cumin. Cook thoroughly for three minutes. Stir in the salsa after removing from heat.

2. Take a microwave-safe dish and place the cut-side down of squash on it. Add two tbsps. of water to the squash. Place the dish (uncovered) inside the microwave and bake for fifteen minutes. Make sure the squash flesh becomes tender.

3. Scrape out the flesh of squash from its shells with a fork. While the turkey mixture is still in the skillet, add the scooped squash flesh to it. Sprinkle remaining salt and then stir well.

4. Take a sheet (baking) and then arrange the squash shells on it. Scoop back the squash mixture into the shells. Top them with cheese. Thoroughly bake for fifteen minutes. Wait until the cheese melts and then top with avocado and lettuce. Serve with extra salsa if desired and enjoy.

Lemon Asparagus Chicken Skillet

Total Prep & Cooking Time: 35 minutes

Yields: Three plates

Nutrition Facts: Calories: 335 | Carbs: 14g | Protein: 36.9g | Fat: 15g | Fiber: 1.6g

Ingredients:

- Two tablespoons of avocado oil
- Half a teaspoon pepper
- One bunch of asparagus
- One-third cup of chicken broth
- One tablespoon of coconut aminos
- One teaspoon each of
  - Salt
  - Arrowroot starch
- One pound of chicken breast, sliced into cubes
- Three garlic cloves, minced
- One lemon juiced

Method:

1. Pour the avocado oil in the skillet and heat it over moderate heat.

2. After the oil starts to bubble out, add the chicken cubes and season with pepper and salt. Cook until the chicken becomes tender (insert the thermometer into the chicken's thickest part and check if it reads a

temperature of 165 degrees F) and then remove the chicken and set it aside.

3. To prepare the asparagus, chop off its thick white base and cut them vertically into halves.

4. Saute the asparagus for seven minutes with more pepper, oil, and salt if needed. They should become soft with a little crisp. Set them aside.

5. Lower the flame and then add the garlic to the skillet. Cook until it gives out the fragrance.

6. One by one, add the arrowroot starch, lemon juice, broth, and the coconut aminos. Stir them for about three minutes until the sauce attains a thickened consistency.

7. Add the asparagus and chicken pieces to the skillet and cook thoroughly for three more minutes.

8. Remove from the heat and top with onion wedges. Season more to satisfy your taste and finally serve it warm.

Note: *This is an allergen-friendly meal that is made with foods that can provide you with the best of protein source and lime that is there to give a touch of acidic flavor. Chicken breast is good-to-go with this dish as it is easy to cook and makes things go smoother. You can omit the pepper part if you are on an AIP diet. Chicken broth is there to add the desired flavor and save the dish from getting thickened.*

Egg Roll in a Bowl

Total Prep & Cooking Time: 30 minutes

Yields: Four servings

Nutrition Facts: Calories: 351 | Carbs: 15.8g | Protein: 38.2g | Fat: 15.8g | Fiber: 2.6g

Ingredients:

For preparing the roll,

- One pound of pork (ground)
- One diced onion (white)
- One teaspoon of ginger (grated)
- Two teaspoons of vinegar (apple cider)
- Two tablespoons each of
  - o Chopped onion (green)
  - o Sesame oil
- Two garlic cloves (diced)
- Twelve ounces of coleslaw mix
- Three tablespoons of coconut aminos

For preparing the sauce (optional),

- A quarter cup of coconut cream
- One teaspoon of vinegar (apple cider)

- Salt
- One tablespoon of coconut aminos
- Two teaspoons of freshly grated ginger

Method:

1. Take a large-sized skillet and cook the pork over moderate flame. Season with salt and pepper. Cook until the pork turns brown and then set it aside. You are recommended to dispose off the fat.

2. Pour some oil in the same skillet and heat over moderate flame. Once the oil starts to boil, add the ginger, garlic, and the onion to it. Cook to turn the onion translucent, and the garlic begins to give fragrance.

3. To the mixture, add the vinegar, coleslaw mix, and the coconut aminos—season with pepper and salt. Stir them properly for about five minutes.

4. Pour back the precooked pork to the skillet and then stir well. Saute the mixture for an additional minute.

5. Transfer the pork to the bowls. Top with the optional sauce and the onion. Serve and enjoy

For preparing the sauce,

1. Combine all ingredients for preparing the sauce and then stir well.

2. Serve the mixture over each bowl.

Note: *Coconut aminos is the substitute for the soy sauce. Avoid using a coleslaw mix that is too much filled with carrots to your dish extra sugary.*

One-pan Chicken Pesto

Total Prep & Cooking Time: 40 minutes

Yields: Three to Four plates of pesto

Nutrition Facts: Calories: 556 | Carbs: 24.5g | Protein: 43g | Fat: 32.5g | Fiber: 4.2g

Ingredients:

For preparing the sheet pan,

- Two pounds of chicken breast (you may substitute with chicken thigh), bone-in
- Two zucchinis (diced)
- One medium-sized red onion (finely chopped)
- Half a tsp. each of
  - Black pepper
  - Sea salt
- Two carrots (thinly sliced into circles)
- One sliced squash (yellow)

For preparing the mint basil pesto,

- One cup each of
  - Arugula
  - Basil (fresh)
- Two tablespoons of fresh mint
- A quarter cup of a freshly juiced lemon
- Half a tsp. of salt
- Half a cup of avocado oil
- One garlic clove (minced and peeled)

Method:

1. Add the ingredients for preparing the pesto into the blender and then process it. Do not turn the blender off until the mixture gets combined thoroughly. After you are done, set the mixture aside.

2. Set the oven at a temperature of 400 degrees F. you will require a baking sheet and a parchment paper. With the parchment paper, line the large-sized baking sheet.

3. Place all ingredients for preparing sheet pan on the sheet evenly. The ingredients must not be crowded. Coat the vegetables and the chicken properly with the pesto. Leave about two tablespoons of pesto for later use.

4. Place the baking sheet on the oven. After every ten minutes, flip the vegetables so that both sides are cooked evenly. Continue cooking for thirty-five minutes. After the said mark, insert a thermometer in the chicken's thickest part. If the reading shows 165 degrees F, then you may stop cooking. It means you have cooked the chicken thoroughly and have tenderized it.

5. Transfer the chicken to the plates. Top each plate with the leftover pesto and serve warm.

Note: An important part to note is that you should prevent overcrowding the pan in which you are cooking. The vegetables must be chopped with even thickness as it will ensure they finish cooking at the same time. The bone-in chicken is recommended as it leads to flavor enhancement and keeps the meat juicy.

BBQ Jackfruit

Total Prep & Cooking Time: 10 minutes

Yields: Two servings

Nutrition Facts: Calories: 471 | Carbs: 83.8g | Protein: 4.9g | Fat: 15.7g | Fiber: 4.7g

Ingredients:

- A can of jackfruit (fourteen ounces)
- Half a teaspoon of salt
- Two teaspoons each of
  - Onion powder
  - Garlic powder
  - Coconut sugar
- Two tablespoons each of
  - Avocado oil
  - Chopped green onion
- A quarter of black pepper
- One teaspoon of chili powder
- Half a cup of BBQ sauce

Method:

1. Remove the excess liquid from the jackfruit can.

2. Place a large-sized pan over a moderate flame. Then add jackfruit and sprinkle some salt, garlic, chili powder, coconut sugar, pepper, and onion. Stir well for three minutes until they soften.

3. Add the BBQ sauce to it and toss the veggies well to coat them with the sauce. Make the vegetables incorporated. Simmer for about three minutes.

4. Transfer the preparation to the plates. Top each plate with onions.

5. Serve warm and enjoy.

Chapter 4: How to Increase Immunity to Prevent Further Relapse?

If you're suffering from Hashimoto's, your thyroid gets inflamed because of the extra stress on your immune system, and as a result, the thyroid hormones are under-produced. You can prevent further relapses of Hashimoto disease and restore the optimal functions of your thyroid by increasing your immunity. You can boost your immunity and restore the function of your thyroid by using a few easy yet proven lifestyle and dietary changes (Premawardhana, 2006).

1. **Repair your gut** – It is essential to repair your gut if you have Hashimoto's. Almost eighty percent of your whole immune system is situated in your digestive system. The intestinal wall should be just a little permeable to allow the nutrients to reach the bloodstream. However, when it gets leaky, bigger molecules can enter your bloodstream and cause chronic inflammation. The immune system detects them as foreign invaders. Some of these invaders are very similar to the blood cells of the body, and so the immune system ends up attacking your thyroid accidentally. Thus, repairing the gut is extremely important. You can do it with the help of the amino acids and nutrients it requires and by eliminating inflammatory foods, parasites, infections, and toxins. You also need to re-inoculate with healthy bacteria and restore the acids and enzymes that are essential for proper digestion.

2. **Tame the toxins** – We are exposed to several hundreds of toxins in our daily lives. Toxins like nitrates, percolates, and mercury can accumulate in your body and impact your thyroid functions as they are chemically similar to iodine. You can, however, eliminate these toxins from your

body and prevent your exposure to them by taking a few necessary steps. Firstly, you need to learn how you are getting exposed to them and then try to minimize your exposure. After that, you can try detox pathways to flush the toxins safely from your body.

3. **Heal your infections** – Bacterial and viral infections can trigger Hashimoto's in various ways. Some common infections often don't show any symptoms. However, they can be tested for and treated.

4. **Relieve your stress** – Your adrenal gland produces and releases a large number of hormones when you're under stress. These signals make the stressor a priority and dismiss other functions, including the production of thyroid hormone and immune response. It can negatively affect your thyroid. Learning how to relieve stress can immensely help prevent the relapse of Hashimoto's. Walking, running, mediation, and deep breathing exercises can all help relieve stress and also prevent you from falling into a state of chronic stress.

PART IV

Be gentle with yourself throughout this process as it will be uncomfortable at times and will require strength. This book will help you through it, as you are not alone. I hope that this book also reminds you that many other people are suffering from the same type of food-related disorders as you are and that you are not alone in that either. This book will take a step-by-step approach, which will make for the highest chance of recovery. If at any time you need to take a break in order to think about the information you have learned, feel free to do so, but make sure you come back to this book quite soon after. Going through this process of recovery can be a lot, but with the right support, it will be possible.

You have already taken the first step in recovery, which is acknowledging that you have an issue. For that, I congratulate you!

What Is Emotional Eating?

Emotional eating occurs when a person suffering from emotional deficiencies of some sort, including lack of affection, lack of connection, or other factors like stress, depression, anxiety, or even general negative feelings like sadness or anger, eats in order to gain comfort from the food they are eating.

Many people find comfort in food. When people experience negative feelings and turn to food consumption in order to reduce their pain or to feel better, this is called emotional eating.

Now, some people do this on occasion like after a breakup or after a bad fight, but when this occurs at least a few times a week, this is when it is considered to have a negative impact on one's life and is when it becomes an issue that needs to be addressed.

What Is Binge Eating?

Binge eating disorder is another disorder that can be seen along with emotional eating. Binge eating disorder is when a person eats much more than a regular amount of food in a single occasion or sitting, and they feel unable to control themselves or to stop themselves. This could also be defined as a compulsion to overeat. In order to be considered a disorder, it has to happen at least two times per week for longer than six months consecutively.

Along with binge eating is overeating, although this is also sometimes seen as a separate disorder altogether. Overeating is when a person eats more than they require in order to sustain life. This occurs when they consume much more than they need in a day, or in a single sitting.

Overeating does not necessarily become binge eating, but it certainly can. Overeating is a general term used to describe the eating disorders that we just defined-Emotional Eating and Binge Eating. Thus, overeating could involve binge eating, food addiction, or other food-related disorders.

In this book, we will be focusing on emotional eating and binge eating, and how you can overcome these two food-related disorders.

What Is Bulimia?

Bulimia is another eating disorder. Bulimia involves binge eating, followed by extreme feelings of shame, guilt, and disdain for oneself and one's body. This is accompanied by intense feelings of body dysmorphia and body image issues, as well as the desire to be "skinnier." Thus, the person will turn to purging- or self-inflicted vomiting in an effort to lose weight and rid themselves of the guilt and shame.

Chapter 1: Understanding Your Food-Related Disorder

In this chapter, we are going to look at these two food-related disorders (binge eating/ bulimia and emotional eating) in much more detail. We will begin by looking at the most common reasons why people suffer from these disorders and will spend some time examining scientific research about why these disorders exist.

Why Do People Eat Emotionally?

The reason that emotional eating occurs is that eating foods that we enjoy makes us feel rewarded on an emotional and physiological level within our brain.

Why Do People Binge Eat?

People binge eat for a very similar reason to the reason why people experience emotional eating. This is because eating foods that we enjoy in terms of taste, smell, texture, and so on, makes us feel rewarded on an emotional and physiological level within our brains.

Throughout the rest of this chapter, we will look more in-depth at these eating disorders in order to give you more information about why they occur and what could cause them.

Scientific Research on Eating Disorders and Why They Exist

You may be asking how food cravings can result from emotional deficiencies and how these two seemingly unrelated things can be considered related. While we have touched on this briefly in this book already, the reason for this is that your body learns, over time, that eating certain foods makes it feel rewarding, positive, and happy for some time after it is ingested. These foods include convenience foods such as those containing processed sugars or salts, fast food, and quick pastries.

When you are sad or worried, your body feels negative and looks for ways to remedy this. Your brain then connects these two facts- that the body does not feel positive and that it wants to find a way to fix this. The brain then decides that eating the foods that make it feel good will remedy the situation. This process happens in the background of your mind without you being aware of it, and it leads you to consciously feel a craving for those specific foods such as sugary snacks or salty fast-food meals. You may not even be aware of why. If you then decide to give in to this craving and eat something like a microwave pizza snack, your body will feel rewarded and happy for a brief period of time. This reinforces to your brain that turning to food in an effort to make yourself feel better emotionally has been successful.

If you end up feeling down and guilty that you ate something that was unhealthy or that you ate too much, your brain will again try and remedy these negative emotions by craving food. This is how a cycle of emotional eating or a cycle of bingeing and purging can begin and continue. This could happen largely in your subconscious without you being any the wiser.

Why Do People Have Bulimia or Other Food Disorders?

Because scientists and psychiatrists understand this process that occurs in the brain, they know that food cravings can indicate emotional deficiencies. While there are other types of cravings that can occur, such as those that pregnant ladies experience, or those that indicate nutrient deficiencies, there are ways to tell that a craving is caused by some type of emotional deficiency.

It begins by determining the foods that a person craves and when they crave them. If every time someone has a stressful situation, they feel like eating a pizza, or if a person who is depressed tends to eat a lot of chocolate, this could indicate emotional eating. As you know by now, emotional eating and bulimia are closely related, and emotional eating can lead to bulimia over time.

If you crave fruit like a watermelon on a hot day, you are likely just dehydrated, and your body is trying to get water from a water-filled fruit that it knows will make it more hydrated. Examining situations like this has led scientists and psychiatrists to explore eating disorders in more depth and determine what types of emotional deficiencies can manifest themselves through food cravings or disordered eating in this way.

In the next chapter, we will look at psychological triggers that can lead to disordered eating.

The Neuroscience of Brain Chemicals and Food As a Reward

Many times, we may see ingredients on the packages of foods we eat, but we aren't really sure of exactly what they are, just that they taste good. In this section, we will take a deeper look at them and what they do to your brain.

Casein is a heavily processed ingredient that is derived from milk. It is processed a few times over and eventually creates milk solids that are concentrated. These milk solids- called Casein are then added into foods like cheese, french fries, milkshakes, and other fast and convenient packaged or fast-foods that contain dairy or dairy products (such as pastries and salad dressings). Casein has been compared to nicotine in its addictive properties. It is often seen in cheese, and this is why there is increasing evidence that people can become, and many are already addicted to cheese. The reason for this is during digestion. When cheese and other foods that contain casein are digested, it is broken down, and one of the compounds that it breaks down into is a compound that is strikingly similar to opioids- the highly addictive substance that is in pain killers.

High fructose corn syrup is surely an ingredient you have heard of before or at least one that you have seen on the packaging of your favorite snacks or quick foods. While this is actually derived from real corn, after it is finished being processed, there is nothing corn-like about it. High fructose corn syrup is essentially the same thing as refined sugar when all is said and done. It is used as a sweetener in foods like soda, cereal, and other sweet and quick foods. The reason why this ingredient is seen so often is that it is much cheaper than using sugar and is much easier to work with. High Fructose Corn Syrup is another common food additive that has been shown to be highly addictive. This substance has been shown to be similar to cocaine in its addictive properties.

MSG stands for Monosodium Glutamate, which sounds a lot like a chemical you may have encountered in science class in college. MSG is added to foods to give it a delicious flavor. It is essentially a very concentrated form of salt. What this does in foods such as fast-food, packaged convenience foods, and buffet-style food is that it gives it that wonderfully salty and fatty flavor that makes us keep coming back for more. Companies put this in food because it comes at an extremely low cost, and the flavor it brings covers up the artificial flavors of all of the other cheap ingredients that are used to make these foods. MSG has been known to block our natural appetite suppressant, which normally kicks in when we have had enough to eat. For this reason, when we are eating foods containing MSG, we do not recognize when we are satiated, and we continue to eat until we are stuffed because it tastes so great.

Chapter 2: Understanding Your Mind

In this chapter, we are going to look at some of the psychological factors that can lead to disordered eating so that you can gain a better understanding of what could have led you to use food as a means of coping.

Psychological and Emotional Triggers

There are several types of emotional deficiencies that can be indicated by disordered eating. We will explore these in detail below in hopes that you will recognize some of the reasons why you may be struggling with an eating disorder.

Childhood Causes

The first example of an emotional deficiency that we will examine is more of an umbrella for various emotional deficiencies. This umbrella term is Childhood Causes. If you think back on your childhood, think about how your relationship with food was cultivated. Maybe you were taught that when you behaved, you received food as a reward. Maybe when you were feeling down, you were given food to cheer you up. Maybe you turned to food when you were experiencing negative things in your childhood. Any of these could cause someone to suffer from emotional eating in their adulthood, as it had become something learned. This type is quite difficult to break as it has likely been a habit for many, many years, but it is possible. When we are children, we learn habits and make associations without knowing it that we often carry into our later lives. While this is no fault of yours, recognizing it as a potential issue is important to make changes.

Covering Up Emotions

Another emotional deficiency that can manifest itself in emotional eating and food cravings is actually the effort to cover up our emotions. Sometimes we would rather distract ourselves and cover up our emotions than to feel them or to face them head-on. In this case, our brain may make us feel hungry in an effort to distract us from the act of eating food. When we have a quiet minute where these feelings or thoughts would pop into our minds, we can cover them up by deciding to prepare food and eat and convince ourselves that we are "too busy" to acknowledge our feelings because we have to deal with our hunger. The fact that it is hunger that arises in this scenario makes it very difficult to ignore and very easy to deem as a necessary distraction since, after all, we do need to eat in order to survive. This can be a problem though, if we are not in need of nourishment, and we are telling ourselves that this is the reason why we cannot deal with our demons or our emotions. If there is something that you think you may be avoiding dealing with or thinking about or if you tend to be very uncomfortable with feelings of unrest, you may be experiencing this type of emotional eating.

Feeling Empty or Bored

When we feel bored, we often decide to eat or decide that we are hungry. This occupies our mind and our time and makes us feel less bored and even feel positive and happy. We also may eat when we are feeling empty. When we feel empty the food will quite literally be ingested in an effort to fill a void, but as we know, the food will not fill a void that is emotional in sort, and this will lead to an unhealthy cycle of trying to fill ourselves emotionally with something that will never actually work. This will lead us to become disappointed every time and continue trying to fill this void with material things like food or purchases. This can also be a general feeling of dissatisfaction with life and feelings of lacking something in your life. Looking deeper into this the next time you feel those cravings will be difficult but will help you greatly in the long term as you will then be able to identify the source of your feelings of emptiness and begin to fill these voids in ways that will be much more effective.

Affection Deficiency

Another emotional deficiency that could manifest itself as food cravings is an affection deficiency. This type of deficiency can be feelings of loneliness, feelings of a lack of love, or feelings of being undesired. If a person has been without an intimate relationship or has recently gone through a breakup, or if a person has not experienced physical intimacy in quite some time, they may be experiencing an affection deficiency. This type of emotional deficiency will often manifest itself in food cravings as we will try to gain feelings of comfort and positivity from the good tasting, drug-like (as we talked about in chapter one) foods they crave.

Low Self-Esteem

Another emotional deficiency that may be indicated by food cravings is a low level of self-esteem. Low self-esteem can cause people to feel down, unlovable, inadequate, and overall negative and sad. This can make a person feel like eating foods they enjoy will make them feel better, even if only for a few moments. Low self-esteem is an emotional deficiency that is difficult to deal with as it affects every area of a person's life, such as their love life, their social life, their career life, and so on. Sometimes people have reported feeling like food was something that was always there for them, and that never left them. While this is true, they will often be left feeling even emptier and lower about themselves after giving into cravings.

Mood

A general low mood can cause emotional eating. While the problem of emotional eating is something that is occurring multiple times per week and we all have general low moods or bad days, if this makes you crave food and especially food of an unhealthy sort, this could become emotional eating. If every time we feel down or are having a bad day, we want to eat food to make ourselves feel better; this is emotional eating. Some people will have a bad day and want a drink at the end of the day, and if this happens every once in a while, it is not necessarily a problem with emotional eating. The more often it happens, the more often it is emotional eating. Further, we do not have to give in to the cravings for it to be considered emotional eating. Experiencing the cravings often and in tandem with negative feelings in the first place is what constitutes emotional eating.

Depression

Suffering from depression also can lead to emotional eating. Depression is a constant low mood for a period of months on end, and this low mood can cause a person to turn to food for comfort and a lift in spirit. This can then become emotional eating in addition to and because of depression.

Anxiety

Having anxiety can lead to emotional eating, as well. There are several types of anxiety, and whether it is general anxiety (constant levels of anxiety), situational anxiety (triggered by a situation or scenario), it can lead to emotional eating. You have likely heard of the term *comfort food* to describe certain foods and dishes. The reason for this is because they are usually foods rich in carbohydrates, fats, and heavy in nature. These foods bring people a sense of comfort. These foods are often turned to when people suffering from anxiety are emotionally eating because these foods help to temporarily ease their anxiety and make them feel calmer and more at ease. This only lasts for a short period of time; however, before their anxiety usually gears up again.

Stress

Stress eating is probably the most common form of emotional eating. While this does not become an issue for everyone experiencing stress, and many people will do so every once in a while, it is a problem for those who consistently turn to food to ease their stress. Some people are always under stress, and they will constantly be looking for ways to ease their stress. Food is one of these ways that people use to make themselves feel better and to take their minds off of their stress. As with all of the other examples we have seen above, this is not a lasting resolution, and it becomes a cycle. Similar to the cycle diagram we saw above, the same can be used for stress except instead of a negative emotion and eating making you feel more down, stress eating can make you feel more stress as you feel like you have done something you shouldn't have which causes you stress, and the cycle ensues.

Recognizing your triggers is important because this will allow you to notice when you may be feeling emotional hunger and when you are feeling actual hunger. If you become hungry, you can look back on your day or on the last hour and determine if any of your triggers were present. If they were, then you will be able to determine that you are likely experiencing emotional hunger, and you can take the appropriate steps instead of giving in to the cravings blindly.

There are many different emotional causes for the cravings we experience. There may be others than those listed above, and these are all valid. A person's emotional eating experience is unique and personal and could be caused by any number of things. You may also experience a combination of emotional deficiencies listed above, or one of those listed above in addition to others. Many of these can overlap, such as anxiety and depression, which are often seen together in a single person. The level of these emotional deficiencies that you experience could indicate the level of emotional eating that you struggle with. Whatever your experience and your struggles though, there is hope of recovery, and this is what the rest of this book will focus on.

Chapter 3: How to Stop Binge Eating, Bulimia, and Emotional Eating

In this chapter, we are going to look at how you can begin to tackle your mind in order to make positive changes for your body and break free from your eating disorder once and for all.

Addressing the Core Wounds

The key to solving these food-related issues is to address your core wounds. Understanding how your mind works will help you to better take care of it. You will be able to recognize your feelings and how they could have come about, and then treat them in a way that will help it to feel better. Bettering your relationship with food and your body will also improve your relationship with your mind. This will then allow you to begin to feed it what it needs, which will, in turn, lead to better cognitive functioning, control over impulses, and decision-making. This will help overall in your relationship with your food, your body, and your mind.

What Are Core Wounds?

As we discussed in the previous chapter, there are several types of emotional deficiencies that can be indicated by disordered eating. Once you have determined which of these emotional deficiencies (or which combination of them) are present in your life, you can begin to look at them in a little more detail. By doing so, you will come upon your core wounds. A core wound is something that you believe to be true about yourself or your life, and it is something that likely came about as a result of a coping mechanism you developed to deal with childhood. For example, this could be something like; the feeling of not being enough, the belief that you are unlovable, or the belief that you are stupid.

How to Address Them

By understanding and addressing your core wounds, you will be able to change your behaviors because of the intricate relationship that exists between your thoughts, your emotions, and your behaviors. By addressing your thoughts and emotions, you will change your behaviors and thus, free yourself from disordered eating. You may be wondering how you can begin to address your core wounds, as it can be difficult to know where to begin.

The first step is learning how to control and change your thoughts, which in turn, leads to changes in your behavior. By taking control of your thoughts and your beliefs, they don't have the opportunity to manifest into unhealthy behaviors such as overeating, turning to food for comfort, or any other unhealthy coping mechanisms that you have developed over the course of your life.

Becoming aware of your own thoughts is the most crucial step in this entire guide, as everything else will fail without it. Paying attention to your thoughts will help you identify what thoughts are going through your mind during an intense emotional moment. By looking deep within, in order to get in touch with your deepest feelings, you will be more likely to succeed in your weight loss and your overall lifestyle improvement.

One great example of how to put this into practice is through the use of journaling. Journaling can help in a process such as this because it can help you to organize your thoughts and feelings and will help you to see visually what is working and what isn't working for you. While we can give tips and examples, every person is different, so to find exactly what works for you, you will have to try some different things and see which techniques help you personally the most and in the best way. Journaling can be about anything like how you feel since beginning a new program, how you feel physically since changing your diet, how you feel emotionally now that you are not reaching for food in order to comfort your emotions and anything along the lines of this.

Positive Self-Talk

Once you have addressed your emotions and your core wounds, you can begin to intervene and change them so that they result in healthier behaviors. You will do this using positive self-talk. Adopting helpful thought processes fosters better emotions overall, which leads to more productive behaviors.

When people have developed unhelpful thinking processes, it is hard to make decisions to benefit their future selves because their thoughts create negative emotions that drive away motivation. This is where something called *positive self-talk* can come in. Positive self-talk can be instrumental in helping you to recover from disordered eating.

What Is Positive Self-Talk?

Many people's minds are controlled by their inner critic. The inner critic shares words with you, such as "You should just give up" Or "What makes you think you'll succeed?" which is rooted in the opposite of positive self-talk- Negative self-talk!

Instead of creating an open space that allows for mistakes, growth, and development, your inner critic causes you to question your worth, which makes it difficult for you to have the positive, growth mindset that is needed to complete tasks and go after things that may be difficult to achieve. In this case, helping your mind to begin using positive self-talk will help you to recover for the long-term.

How to Use Positive Self-Talk?

Below are several ways that you can begin to use positive self-talk. Over time, your mind will get used to thinking in this way, and you will find it much easier to do.

1. Remind yourself

Bad habits are built through many years, and no amount of willpower can undo a lifetime of bad habits, such as a strong inner critic that uses negative self-talk. By rewiring your brain to minimize the amount of negativity you feel in the first place, you will eventually get used to filling your mind with positive thoughts instead of negative ones.

2. Stop the automatic process of negativity

Often times, if the person had just paid attention to their thought process, they would be able to catch themselves before their mind automatically spiraled to a place of complete de-motivation. By catching yourself before you get there, you can prevent yourself from falling into your negative thought patterns that are limiting you and holding you back.

3. Find positive influences

Surrounding yourself with people that can encourage you and foster positivity will also change your inner-critic's opinion. Often times, hearing positive compliments from other people hold a heavier weight in the eyes of your inner-critic compared to you telling your inner-critic the same thing. Try spending time with people who are supportive of your goals and the changes that you are looking to make in your life. It will make your journey a little bit easier.

4. Limit Negative Influences

By limiting the negative influences in your life, you are making a statement to yourself that you place importance on preserving your mental health. When you remove negative influences and limit your exposure to things or people that make you feel negative, you are prioritizing yourself, and this is a great way to practice self-care.

5. Practice a gratitude exercise

This is a great exercise to remind yourself of everything that you love and appreciate about yourself and your life. Take time to write down all of the things that you love about yourself and about your life. This will remind you of all of the positivity surrounding you and will serve to uplift you.

Chapter 4: Making Healthier Decisions Using Intuitive

Eating

This chapter will provide you with a solid foundation of knowledge on which to build your new lifestyle. We will look at how intuitive eating can be the answer to all of your struggles and help you to find recovery.

Making Good Choices

As we discussed in the previous chapter, making good choices begins with self-exploration and a deep look into your core wounds. Once you have done this, you can begin to make decisions that are positive for your health and your life, and over time these will become more and more habitual. We are going to spend this chapter looking at some of the ways that you can begin to make good choices related to food and eating.

How to Begin Making Good Choices Using Intuitive Eating

One great way to make good choices when it comes to food is by using something called intuitive eating. Below, I will define intuitive eating for you and give you some insight into how this can change your life.

What Is Intuitive Eating?

Intuitive eating is a new perspective from which to view how you feed your body. This style of eating puts you in control, instead of following a list of pre-designed guidelines about when and what to eat. Intuitive eating instead encourages you to listen to your body and the signals it sends you about what, how much, and when to eat. This ensures that you are giving your body exactly what it needs when it needs it, instead of forcing it into a specific kind of diet.

Intuitive eating does not limit any specific foods and does not require you to stick to certain foods exclusively. Instead, it encourages you to learn as much as you can about what your body is telling you and follow its signals.

The two main components of the intuitive eating philosophy are the following; eat when you are hungry and stop eating when you are satiated. This may seem like a no-brainer, but in today's societies, we are very far from eating in an intuitive way, as odd as it may seem. With so many diet trends and numerous "rules" for how you should and should not eat, it can be difficult to put these ideas aside and let your body guide you exclusively.

Intuitive Eating and Hunger

Before we begin looking at the specifics of intuitive eating, we will look at the different types of hunger and how you can tell them apart. This will help you to distinguish when you are hungry and when you may be turning to food to soothe your emotional state.

Real hunger is when our body needs nutrients or energy and is letting us know that we should replenish our energy soon. This happens when it has been a few hours since our last meal when we wake up in the morning, or after a lot of strenuous activity like a long hike. Our body uses hunger to signal to us that it is in need of more energy and that if it doesn't get it soon, it will begin to use our stored energy as fuel. While there is nothing wrong with our body using its stored fuel, it can be used as a sign to us that we should eat shortly in order to replenish these stores. Perceived Hunger is when we think we are hungry, but our body doesn't actually require any more energy or for the stores to be replenished. This can happen for a number of reasons, including an emotional deficiency, a negative mental state, or the occurrence of a psychological trigger.

The philosophy behind intuitive eating is that if you wait until you are too hungry before eating, you will be much more likely to overeat or to binge eat. This is because, by this time, you be feeling ravenous instead of mildly hungry. If instead, you choose to adhere to your hunger and eat when your body tells you that it needs sustenance, you will be much more likely to eat just the right amount. As a result, your body will be satisfied rather than completely stuffed, and instead of feeling shameful and angry that you have eaten, you can feel happy that you have provided your body with what it needed. This requires you to listen to and respect what your body is telling you and then provide it with nutrients in order for it to keep working hard for you!

The Benefits of Intuitive Eating

One of the reasons that intuitive eating is such a successful and cherished form of eating is that it allows the body to lead the mind in the right direction when it comes to seeking out its needs. Below, we will look at the benefits of letting your body guide your eating choices.

- Allows the body to get what it needs

Did you know that your cravings could actually be giving you much more information than you give them credit for?
A craving is an intense longing for something (in this case food), that comes about intensely and feels urgent. In our case, that longing is for s a very specific type of food. When we have cravings for certain foods, it can actually mean more than what it seems.

While you may think that a craving is an indication of hunger or of a desire for the taste of a certain food, it may actually indicate that your body is low on certain vitamins or minerals. As a result, your body seeks out a certain food that it thinks will provide it with this vitamin or mineral. This reaches your consciousness in the form of an intense craving. In this case, the body is trying to help itself by telling you what to eat. For this reason, understanding your cravings could help you give your body exactly what it is longing for.

For example, if you are craving juice or pop or other sugary drinks like this, consider that you might actually be dehydrated and, therefore, thirsty. Sometimes we see drinks in our fridge, and since we are thirsty, we really want them. Next time you are craving a sugary drink, try having a glass of water first, then wait a few minutes and see if you are still craving that Coca-Cola. You may not want it anymore once your thirst is quenched.

If you are craving meat, you may feel like you want some fried chicken or a hot dog. This can indicate a deficit of iron or protein. The best sources of protein are chicken breast cooked in the oven, and iron is best received from spinach, oysters, or lentils. If you think you may not like these foods, there are many different ways to prepare them, and you can likely find a way that you like.

- Prevents overeating

It can be hard to know how much to eat and when you have had enough to eat without letting yourself eat too much. Sometimes people will eat until the point that they begin to feel completely full. Many times, we keep eating until we become stuffed, even to the point of making ourselves feel physically ill. Intuitive eating will help you to avoid this, as this kind of eating encourages you to give your body what it needs in order to take great care of it. Stuffing your body until it is too full is not what your body is asking for, and once you become accustomed to listening to your body's needs, you will know when it is time to stop.

- Helps you break free from self-judgment

intuitive eating will help you to finally make peace with your body and yourself as a whole. It does this by showing you that your body has needs and that there is no shame in tending to these needs, as long as you do so in a healthy way.

You cannot fully embrace and practice intuitive eating if you have those nagging feelings of self-judgment each time you take a bite of food or decide that you are going to eat lunch when you are hungry. For this reason, in order to practice intuitive eating, you must understand that feeding your body is an act of compassion for yourself and that this does not need to come with self-judgment.

- It is inclusive, not exclusive

One of the great things about this style of eating is that it is not founded on restricting a person's intake of certain foods or allowing only a small variety of foods.

Diets like this are extremely hard to transition to and are hard to maintain for a long period of time. Intuitive eating is about including as many natural whole foods as you wish, while also ensuring that you are consuming enough of all of your nutrients. With this style of eating, you can eat whatever you wish, whenever you wish. This makes it much easier to stick with this type of diet and reduces the chances of falling off after a short period of time due to cravings or intense hunger. It does not restrict calories or reduce your intake greatly, which makes it easier to handle than a traditional diet for many people. It feels natural to eat in this way, which makes it effective.

Chapter 5: Intuitive Eating Part 2

In this chapter, we are going to continue our examination of intuitive eating by looking at some more specific details related to this diet, as well as how to make it a regular part of your life.

How to Make Intuitive Eating Part of Your Life

One of the best ways to make this type of eating a part of your life is to practice it with intention. This is especially important when you are just beginning. Each time you feel a pang of hunger or a compulsion to eat, take a minute to examine your inner world. By doing this, you will get your mind and body accustomed to working together. In addition, do the same after you eat. By doing these two things, you will be able to ensure that you are eating when hungry and stopping when satisfied.

When you finish eating a meal, rank your level of fullness on a scale of 1 to 10, 1 being extremely hungry and 10 being extremely stuffed. This will help you to determine if you are successfully stopping when you are satisfied and not overeating.

It is also important that you learn how to deal with your emotions and feelings in an effective way without using food. Using the techniques that you have learned in this book, you will be able to address your inner demons, which will make space for you to listen to your body and its needs.

As you know by now, listening to your body, your emotions and your mind is extremely important when it comes to practicing intuitive eating. As long as you remember this, you will be well on your way to becoming a lifelong intuitive eater.

What Kind of Foods Should You Choose?

Fish is a great way to get healthy fats into your diet. Certain fish are very low in carbohydrates but high in good fats, making them perfect for a healthy diet. They also contain minerals and vitamins that will be good for your health. Salmon is a great fish to eat, as it is versatile and delicious. Many fish also include essential fatty acids that we can only get through our diet. Other fish that are good for you include:

- Sardines
- Mackerel
- Herring
- Trout
- Albacore Tuna

Meat and Poultry make up a large part of most Americans' diets. Meats and poultry that are fresh and not processed do not include any carbohydrates and contain high levels of protein. Eating lean meats helps to maintain your strength and muscle mass and gives you energy for hours. Grass-fed meats, in particular, are rich in antioxidants.

Eggs are another amazing, protein-filled food. Eggs help your body to feel satiated for longer and also keeps your blood sugar levels consistent, which is great for overall health. The whole egg is good for you, as the yolk is where the nutrients are. The cholesterol found within egg yolks also has been demonstrated to lower your risk of getting diseases like heart diseases, despite what most people think. Therefore, do not be afraid of the egg yolk!

Legumes are a great source of protein as well as fiber, and there are many different types to choose from. These include the following:

- All sorts of beans including black beans, green beans, and kidney beans
- Peas
- Lentils of all colors
- Chickpeas
- Peas

Examples of fruits that you can eat include the following:

- Citrus fruits such as oranges, grapefruits, lemons, and limes
- Melons of a variety of sorts
- Apples
- Bananas
- Berries including strawberries, blueberries, blackberries, raspberries and so on
- Grapes

Vegetables are a great source of energy and nutrients, and they include a wide range of naturally occurring vivid colors which should all be included in your diet.

- Carrots
- Broccoli and cauliflower

- Asparagus

- Kale

- All sorts of peppers including hot peppers, bell peppers

- Tomatoes

- Root vegetables (that are a good source of healthy, complete carbohydrates) such as potatoes, sweet potatoes, all types of squash, and beets.

Seeds are another great source of nutrients, vitamins, and minerals, and they are very versatile. These include the following:

- Sesame seeds

- Pumpkin seeds

- Sunflower seeds

- Hemp, flax and chia seeds are all especially good for your health

Nuts are a great way to get protein if you are choosing not to eat meat or if you are vegan. They also are packed with nutrients. Some examples are below.

- Almonds

- Brazil Nuts

- Cashews

- Macadamia nuts

- Pistachios

- Pecans

There are some **healthy fats** that are essential components of any person's diet, as the beneficial compounds that they contain cannot be made by our bodies; thus, we rely solely on or diet to get them. These compounds are Omega-3 Fatty

Acids, monounsaturated and polyunsaturated fats. Below are some healthy sources of these compounds:

- Avocados
- Healthy, plant-based oils including olive oil and canola oil
- Hemp, chia and flax seeds
- Walnuts

When it comes to carbohydrates, these should be consumed in the form of **whole grains**, as they are high in fiber, which will help to prevent overeating. Whole grains also include essential minerals- those that we can only get from our diet just like those essential compounds found in healthy fats. These essential minerals are selenium, magnesium, and copper. Sources of these whole grains include the following:

- Quinoa
- Rye, Barley, buckwheat
- Whole grain oats
- Brown rice
- Whole grain bread can be hard to find these days in the grocery store, as many brown breads disguise themselves as whole grain when, in fact, they are not. However, there are whole grain breads if you take the time to look at the ingredients list.

Nutrients You Need and How to Get Them

In this section, we are going to look at the most beneficial nutrients for your body and where/ how you can find them. This will help you to decide which foods to include in your diet so that you can ensure you are getting all of the nutrients that your body needs.

1. Omega-3 Fatty Acids

Some vitamins and nutrients are called "essential nutrients." Omega-3 Fatty Acids are an example of this type of nutrient. They are called essential nutrients because they cannot be made by our bodies; thus, they must be eaten in our diets. These fatty acids are a very specific type of fatty acid, and this type, in particular, is the most essential and the most beneficial for our brains and bodies.

They have numerous effects on the brain, including reducing inflammation (which reduces the risk of Alzheimer's) and maintaining and improving mood and cognitive function, including specifically memory. Omega-3's have these greatly beneficial effects because of the way that they act in the brain, which is what makes them so essential to our diets. Omega-3 Fatty Acids increase the production of new nerve cells in the brain by acting specifically on the nerve stem cells within the brain, causing new and healthy nerve cells to be generated.

Omega-3 fatty acids can be found in fish like salmon, sardines, black cod, and herring. It can also be taken as a pill-form supplement for those who do not eat fish or cannot eat enough of it. It can also be taken in the form of a fish oil supplement like krill oil.

Omega-3 is by far the most important nutrient that you need to ensure you are ingesting because of the numerous benefits that come from it, both in the brain and in the rest of the body. While supplements are often a last step when it comes to trying to include something in your diet, for Omega-3's, the benefits are too great to potentially miss by trying to receive all of it from your diet.

Magnesium

Magnesium is beneficial for your diet, as it also helps you to maintain strong bones and teeth. Magnesium and Calcium are most effective when ingested together, as Magnesium helps in the absorption of calcium. It also helps to reduce migraines and is great for calmness and relieving anxiety. Magnesium can be found in leafy green vegetables like kale and spinach, as well as fruits like bananas and raspberries, legumes like beans and chickpeas, vegetables like peas, cabbage, green beans, asparagus, and brussels sprouts, and fish like tuna and salmon.

Calcium

Calcium is beneficial for the healthy circulation of blood, and for maintaining strong bones and teeth. Calcium can come from dairy products like milk, yogurt, and cheese. It can also be found in leafy greens like kale and broccoli and sardines.

Chapter 6: How to Make These New Choices a Habit

Now that you have learned a wealth of information about intuitive eating, we are going to look at some strategies that you can use to make these new, healthy choices a habit. This will take time, but by employing these strategies, you will surely find success.

Healthy Thinking Patterns

In this section, we will look at a real-life example of dealing with challenges to demonstrate healthy thinking patters when it comes to intuitive eating.

Let's say you are trying to focus on healthy eating, and you find that you have had trouble doing so. Maybe you ate a cupcake, or maybe you had a soda at breakfast. From the perspective of traditional diet mentality, this would become a problem for the diet, and this would become a problem in your mind as well. You would likely be beating yourself up and feeling terrible about the choice you have made.

Let's look at this example in more detail. It is very important to avoid beating yourself up or self-judging for falling off the wagon. This may happen sometimes. What we need to do though, is to focus not on the fact that it has happened, but on how we are going to deal with and react to it. There are a variety of reactions that a person may have to this type of situation. We will examine the possible reactions and their pros and cons below:

- You may feel as though your progress is ruined and that you might as well begin again another time. This could lead you to go back to your old ways and keep you from trying again for quite some time. This could happen many times, over and over again, and each time you slip up, you decide that you might as well give up this time and try again, but each time it ends the same.

- You may fall off of your plan and tell yourself that this day is a write-off and that you will begin again the next day. The problem with this method is that continuing the rest of the day as you would have before you decided to make a change will make it so that the next day is like beginning all over again, and it will be very hard to begin again. You may be able to begin again the next day, and it could be fine, but you must be able to really motivate yourself if you are going to do this. Knowing that you have fallen off before makes it so that you may feel down on yourself and feel as though you can't do it, so beginning again the next day is very important.

- The third option, similar to the previous case, you may fall off, but instead of deciding that the day is a write-off, you tell yourself that the entire week is a write-off, and you then decide that you will pick it up again the next week. This will be even harder than starting again the next day as multiple days of eating whatever you like will make it very hard to go back to making the healthy choices again afterward.

- After eating something that you wish you hadn't (and that wasn't a healthy choice), you decide not to eat anything for the rest of the day so that you don't eat too many calories or too much sugar, and decide that the next day you will start over again. This is very difficult on the body as you are going to be quite hungry by the time the evening rolls around. Instead of forgiving yourself, you are punishing yourself, and it will make it very hard not to reach for chips late at night when you are starving and feeling down.

- The fifth and final option is what you should do in this situation.

This option is the best for success and will make it the most likely that you will succeed long-term. If you fall off at lunch, let's say, because you are tired and, in a rush, and you just grab something from a fast-food restaurant instead of going home for lunch or buying something at the grocery store to eat, this is how we will deal with it. Firstly, you will likely feel like you have failed and may feel quite down about having made an unhealthy choice. Now instead of starving for the rest of the day or eating only lettuce for dinner, you will put this slip up at lunch behind you, and you will continue your day as if it never happened. You will eat a healthy dinner as you planned, and you will continue on with the plan. You will not wait until tomorrow to begin again; you will continue as you would if you had made that healthy choice at lunch. The key to staying on track is being able to bounce back. The people who can bounce back mentally are the ones who will be most likely to succeed. You will need to maintain a positive mental state and look forward to the rest of the day and the rest of the week in just the same way as you did before you had a slip-up. One bad meal out of the entire week is not going to ruin all of your progress and recovering from emotional eating is largely a mental game. It is more mental than anything else, so we must not underestimate the role that our mindset plays in our success or failure.

By using this type of thinking, you will set yourself up for success and will not fall off of your plan completely after one slip up.

Healthy Lifestyle Changes

One important way to ensure that these healthy choices stick for good is by changing some aspects of your lifestyle. By doing this, you will reduce the chances of slipping up by eliminating them altogether. For example, you can change the way you approach the grocery store.

When you are entering the grocery store, it is important that you change a few things about the way you shop, in order to set yourself up for success. This is especially important when you are just beginning your intuitive eating practice, as it will be challenging for you to enter the grocery store and avoid cravings and temptations.

The first thing to keep in mind when grocery shopping for a new diet is to enter with a list. By doing this, you are giving yourself a guide to follow, which will prevent you from picking up things that you are craving or things that you feel like eating in that moment.

One of the biggest things to keep in mind when beginning a new eating practice like intuitive eating is to avoid shopping when you are hungry. This will make you reach for anything and everything that you see. By entering the grocery store when you are satiated or when you have just eaten, you will be able to stick to your list and avoid falling prey to temptations.

If you treat your grocery shopping experience like a treasure hunt, you will be able to cross things off of the list one at a time without venturing to the parts of the grocery store that will prove to be a challenge for you to resist. If you are making healthy eating choices, you will likely be spending most of your time at the perimeter of the grocery store. This is where the whole, plant-based foods are located. By doing this, and entering with a list, you will be able to avoid the middle aisles where the processed, high-sugar temptation foods are all kept.

Having a plan is key when it comes to succeeding in learning new habits and employing a new lifestyle. This plan can be as detailed as you wish, or it can simply come in the form of a general overview. I recommend you start with a more detailed plan in the beginning as you ease into things.

As everyone is different, you may be the type of person who likes lots of lists and plans, or you may be the type of person who doesn't, but for everyone, beginning with a plan and following it closely for the first little while is best. For example, this plan can include things like what you will focus on each week, what you will reduce your intake of, and what you will try to achieve in terms of the mental work involved.

Once you have come up with a general plan for your new lifestyle and how you want it to look, you can then begin laying out more specific plans.

Planning your individual meals will make it much easier for you when you get home from work or when you wake up tired in the morning and need to pack something for your lunch.

You can plan your meals out a week in advance, two weeks or even a month if you wish. You can post this up on your fridge, and each day you will know exactly what you are eating, with no thinking required. This way, there won't be a chance for you to consider ordering a pizza or heating up some chicken fingers because you will already know exactly what you are going to make. By approaching your new style of eating in this way, you can make this transition easier on yourself and ensure success every step of the way.

30-Day Meal Plan

The following 30-day meal plan includes a variety of meals that you can make in order to keep your first thirty days interesting and tasty!

Day 1

- Breakfast:

Coffee

Feta, mushroom and spinach, omelet.

- Lunch:

Oven-baked tempeh with broccoli and cauliflower rice.

- Dinner:

Chicken Caesar salad- tofu and romaine lettuce, parmesan

Day 2

- Breakfast:

Unsweetened yogurt with a mix of some berries such as strawberries, raspberries, and some seeds like flax seeds and chia seeds, and nuts like sliced almonds and walnuts.

- Lunch:

A healthy lunch-time salad with avocado, cheese, grape tomatoes, and a variety of nuts and seeds like spicy pumpkin seeds. Add a salad dressing on top such as blue cheese or ranch dressing, or a homemade one using olive oil and garlic.

- Dinner:

Chicken breast with onions and a homemade tomato sauce. Served alongside some grilled zucchini or eggplant.

Day 3

- Breakfast:

A no sugar added full fat Greek yogurt bowl with seeds, nuts and berries.

1 Cup of coffee

- Lunch:

Make your own lunch box, including firm tofu or meat of some sort, raw tomatoes, any type of cheese cubes that you wish, pickles, a hard-boiled egg, vegetables such as celery, carrots, radishes or zucchini, nuts for protein and fat such as walnuts, or almonds, homemade guacamole (avocado, onion, garlic, jalapeno).

- Dinner:

Grilled portobello, grilled eggplant and grilled zucchini as well as cherry tomatoes sautéed in extra virgin olive oil with garlic. Served with rice and protein such as pork or chicken.

Day 4

- Breakfast:

Coffee

Homemade mushroom & Spinach Frittata, including any vegetables that you wish such as bell peppers and onion.

- Lunch:

Cream cheese with cucumber slices for dipping.

Hard-boiled egg

Meatballs with sweet and sour sauce

- Dinner

Bacon, Avocado, Lettuce, Tomato panini.

Day 5

- Breakfast:

Egg Salad with lettuce, cucumber and whole grain bread.

- Lunch:

Homemade guacamole (avocado, onion, garlic, jalapeno, lime juice) with raw zucchini slices for dipping.

Hard-boiled egg

Tuna

- Dinner:

Cauliflower gratin (cheese, cauliflower, onion, garlic and so on)

As well as chopped lettuce drizzled with Caesar Dressing

Day 6

- Breakfast:

Coffee with heavy cream or coconut oil.

Celery sticks, dipped in peanut or Almond Butter

- Lunch:

Leftover cauliflower gratin

As well as chopped lettuce drizzled with Caesar Dressing

- Dinner:

Cooked or raw broccoli with grated cheese on top

Steak seared in olive oil

Day 7

- Breakfast:

Pancakes with fresh fruits

Black Coffee

- Lunch:

Cold pasta salad with fresh vegetables

Feta and Tomato Meatballs

Raw fresh spinach

- Dinner:

Spicy Spaghetti Squash Casserole

Fresh spinach, raw or cooked with 1 Tbsp ranch dressing drizzled on top.

Day 8

- Breakfast

Smoothie

- Lunch

Tempeh meatballs with guacamole and raw vegetable salad

- Dinner

Rice noodle stir fry with your choice of vegetables and tofu

Day 9

- Breakfast

Omelet cooked in coconut oil with cheese, onions, bell pepper and tomatoes

- Lunch

Tofu scramble with vegetables such as spinach and mushrooms and cheese

- Dinner

Curry with chicken, rice and coconut milk sauce with hot chili paste

Day 10

- Breakfast

Full fat yogurt unsweetened with berries, chia seeds, flax seeds

- Lunch

Cobb salad with boiled egg, vegetables of your choice, tofu, tempeh or chicken and Caesar dressing

- Dinner

Homemade pizza with your choice of toppings

Day 11

- Breakfast

Smoothie with chia seeds and flax seeds, berries and plant-based protein powder, as well as plant-based milk

- Lunch

Salad with tofu or boiled egg, olive oil dressing, spinach and diced vegetables

- Dinner

Vegetarian frittata using coconut oil, spinach, mushroom, cheese, bell peppers and tomato

Day 12

- Breakfast

Greek yogurt no sugar added with nuts and seeds

- Lunch

Homemade tacos with your choice of toppings, including ground turkey

- Dinner

Macaroni and cheese with crumbled roasted bread crumbs on top

Day 13

- Breakfast

Whole grain oats with no sugar added, nuts, flax and chia seeds as well as heavy cream and a plant-based nut butter.

- Lunch

Lettuce wraps with curried tofu and grilled eggplant and zucchini

- Dinner

Homemade burritos filled with crumbled, seasoned meat of your choice, sour cream, guacamole and diced tomatoes

Day 14

- Breakfast

Greek yogurt no sugar added with nuts and seeds

- Lunch

Avocado egg bowls with bacon

- Dinner

Fried rice with your choice of vegetables, scrambled egg and tofu

Day 15

- Breakfast

Coffee with heavy cream and no sugar added

- Lunch

Carrots with guacamole, cottage cheese with nuts and seeds and homemade baked zucchini chips with olive oil drizzle

- Dinner

Egg Salad with Lettuce Wraps

Day 16

- Breakfast

Pancakes with no sugar added maple syrup

- Lunch

Vegetarian egg quiche with spinach and mushroom

- Dinner

Broccoli salad with onion, a cheese of your choice, creamy ranch dressing, almonds and walnuts sliced, as well as some avocado and tofu cubes

Day 17

- Breakfast

Potato hash browns fried in olive oil, sunny side up egg and tempeh "bacon" with a side of grilled tomatoes

- Lunch

Avocadoes stuffed with cauliflower "taco meat", homemade salsa with tomatoes and herbs, sour cream, and grated cheese

- Dinner

Cooked or raw broccoli

Small amount of butter that can be added to the broccoli for taste

Grated cheese on top that can also be added to the broccoli

With steak seared in olive oil

Day 18

- Breakfast

Shakshuka with eggs, tomatoes and parsley

- Lunch

Grilled zucchini roll ups with tomato and cheese

- Dinner

Coconut milk curry with rice, bell peppers and tofu

Day 19

- Breakfast

Breakfast smoothie with berries, no sugar added and full fat milk

- Lunch

Broccoli and cheese fritters with homemade hummus to dip and a side of carrots, celery and cucumber for dipping

- Dinner

Cobb salad including hard-boiled egg, ham cubes, your choice of vegetables and an olive oil or ranch dressing

Day 20

- Breakfast

Spinach and mushroom frittata

- Lunch

Sandwich with scrambled eggs, spinach and mushrooms cooked in olive oil and topped with lettuce, tomato or any other fillings or toppings you wish to include. Finally, add a homemade creamy avocado sauce with avocado, cilantro, pepper and salt and some sour cream.

- Dinner

Rice risotto with cheese, vegetable broth and mushrooms

Day 21

- Breakfast

Unsweetened yogurt with a mix of berries such as strawberries, raspberries, and some seeds like flax seeds and chia seeds, and nuts like sliced almonds and walnuts.

- Lunch

Caesar salad- dressing with no sugar added

Raw vegetables, mixed greens and tempeh

- Dinner

Cauliflower gratin- cheese, cauliflower and choice of vegetables

Day 22

- Breakfast

Hash browns fried in olive oil, sunny side up egg and bacon with a side of grilled tomatoes

- Lunch

Stuffed half zucchini with feta cheese, tomato sauce (no sugar added) and herbs for topping

- Dinner

Mashed potatoes using whole milk and cheese, with grilled eggplant and mushrooms

Day 23

- Breakfast

Nut butter smoothie with yogurt, nut butter, flax seeds, chia seeds

- Lunch

Pan fried steak seasoned with herbs and olive oil, paired with

A spinach salad with raw vegetables of choice and no sugar added Caesar dressing

- Dinner

Cauliflower pasta salad with celery, spinach, onions, and walnuts

Day 24

- Breakfast

Feta, mushroom and Spinach, omelet

Coffee

- Lunch

Coleslaw with a creamy cilantro dressing, carrots, cabbage, celery, tomato and herbs for topping

- Dinner

Crispy tofu cubes with zucchini noodles and a homemade peanut sauce

Day 25

- Breakfast

No bake protein bars

Coffee with no sugar added

- Lunch

Roasted tomatoes with goat cheese, spinach, cilantro and olive oil & balsamic drizzle

- Dinner

Eggplant and zucchini "French fries" with olive oil and crispy tofu cubes

Baked chicken breast

Day 26

- Breakfast

Pancakes with no sugar added maple syrup, full fat Greek yogurt and berries for topping

- Lunch

Low carb broccoli cheese soup with crispy cauliflower on the side

- Dinner

Curried rice with choice of vegetables, such as bell peppers and broccoli

Day 27

- Breakfast

Breakfast salad with scrambled egg, avocado, mixed greens, grilled tomatoes and cheese

- Lunch

Fried goat cheese with roasted red peppers, spinach and olive oil drizzle

- Dinner

Spicy Spaghetti Squash Casserole

Fresh spinach, raw or cooked with ranch dressing drizzled on top

Day 28

- Breakfast

Full fat yogurt unsweetened with berries, chia seeds, flax seeds

- Lunch

Vegetarian chili with tomato, sour cream, a variety of beans and tomatoes

- Dinner

Zucchini spiral pasta noodles with creamy yogurt avocado sauce

Day 29

- Breakfast

Cauliflower "bread" grilled cheese sandwich (similar to cauliflower crust pizza but made as a grilled cheese sandwich instead.

- Lunch

Green beans with mushrooms and tomatoes with a chicken breast on the side

- Dinner

Grape tomato marinara on pasta noodles with parmigiano Reggiano cheese and fresh cracked pepper.

Day 30

- Breakfast

Egg taco shells filled with choice of vegetables

- Lunch

Baked crispy tofu steaks with a sesame seed crust on a bed of zucchini strips and spinach

- Dinner

Baked Spaghetti squash filled with roasted tomatoes and eggplant, topped with melted, crispy cheese

Chapter 7: What to Do Next

As you take all of this information forth with you, it may seem overwhelming to begin applying this to your own life. Remember, life is a process, and you do not need to expect perfection from yourself right away. By taking the first step- reading this book, you are already on your way to changing your life. If you fall off and find that you are back to your old ways, try to find inspiration in the pages of this book once again. If you find that you are unable to find success on your own, there is no shame in seeking professional help. There are many people who are trained professionals in dealing with disordered eating and who can serve as a mentor or a guide for you as you navigate this challenge.

How To Seek Help If It Becomes Uncontrollable?

Understanding and accepting that you need help is the first step to recovery. By reading this book, you have taken this step. If you need further help, there is no shame in accepting this fact. There are many ways to seek help for disordered eating, depending on the level of help that you need. Below is a list of ways that you can seek help, ordered from least to most help.

- Online resources
- Support System
- Support Group
- Group counseling
- Anonymous online counseling or telephone counseling
- One on One counseling

- Talk therapy
- Rehab centers

Counseling or Therapy

Talking therapies are very effective treatments for disordered eating. The things that people learn in therapy gives them the insight and skills in order to feel better and tackle their eating disorder, as well as to prevent it from coming back in the future.

One example of talk therapy is Cognitive Behavioral Therapy or CBT. The way that cognitive behavioral therapy works is by putting an emphasis on the relationship between a person's thoughts, emotions, and behaviors. The theory behind this is that when a person changes any one of these components, change will be initiated in the others. The goal of CBT is to help a person decrease negative thoughts or the amount of worry they experience in order to increase their overall quality of life.

If you think that this is something you would benefit from, please reach out to your local resources to find out more.

PART V

Chapter 1: Chronic Acid Reflux & Its Serious health Implications

Acid reflux is the result of abundant backflow of acid for your stomach into the esophagus. Anatomically, when your lower esophageal sphincter (LES) becomes weakened by, among many causal factors, continually consuming a high diet, acid can flow back into your esophagus causing acid reflux. Consequently, there are numerous symptoms that are spawned by acid reflux including, most notoriously, heartburn and indigestion. While high acidity in the gut is common for everybody and is often devoid of serious health concerns if occurring on a minimal basis, serious health concerns can develop if high acidity can persist for a prolonged period of time. If left unattended and without measures of control put in place, in many instances, these health issues will lead to hospitalization or even death.

In the most serious cases, chronic long-term heartburn, known as Gastroesophageal Reflux Disease (GERD), Barett's esophagus and esophageal problems can arise due to uncontrolled and unaddressed chronic acidity. Some of these most serious ailments are the remnants of years of neglecting the symptoms of acid reflux, particularly after big meals. Over time, the backflow of acid from your stomach damages your esophagus causing erosion of the layers lining the walls of the organ. This inflammation often leads to very painful swelling in esophagus called esophagitis and is accompanied by a painful swallowing feeling. In addition, esophageal ulcers are the most common ailment of an inflamed esophagus. In fact, GERD is the main cause of these ulcers in the lining of the esophagus. Moreover, painful swallowing, nausea, chest pain contribute to a lack of sleep which perpetuates many of these symptoms simplify virtue of that fact that your body is not getting the required rest to overcome these symptoms. As soon as these symptoms arise, be sure to consult a doctor too so that you can be prescribed medication to treat the symptoms before they grow into more serious, persistent conditions. Acquiring medial intervention is especially important when dealing with an ulcer; indeed, ulcers are extremely harmful to the lining of your organ and can be incredibly persistent if left unattended and given time to grow.

Even more, if your highly acidic diet remains the same as before the ulcer, this contributing factor will only enhance the growth of your ulcer and some of your other symptoms. Over time, the scarring of the lining within your esophagus will lead to scar tissue build up, thereby narrowing the esophagus altogether. Swallowing food and drinks will be made much more difficult as a result and may require a surgical procedure to expand the esophagus. These narrow areas of your esophagus are called strictures, and will likely lead to dangerous weight loss and or dehydration. Avoiding a procedure through immediate medical treatment of high acidity is clearly the preferred approach; but once these strictures block your esophageal pathways, a surgical procedure will be required.

Another common ailment of high acidity that affects many people is Barret's esophagus. Specifically, around 10%-15 of people who suffer from GERD will begin to also develop this painful condition, which results in dangerous changes in cells due to excess stomach acid. Thankfully, less than 1% of those who suffer from Barret's esophagus will actually develop esophageal cancer. If intervened early enough in the process, doctors are able to remove any of these abnormally developed cells through a procedure known as an endoscopy, whereby doctors will insert a flexible tube accompanied by a small camera into your esophagus. However, those who have GERD are at a, albeit slightly, increased risk of developing esophageal cancer. Even still, be sure to consult a doctor as soon as your symptoms reach a persistently painful level so that proactive measures and treatment can be implemented to quell your pain, and inhibit the growth of cancer cells.

If there is a long history of esophageal cancer in your family, you will be at an increased risk of developing this cancer as well, especially if you attain medical treatment after a prolonged period of time experiencing symptoms of high acidity. If you are aware of having a family history of esophageal cancer, make sure to ask your doctor for a regular endoscopy to find and mitigate the growth of improper cells. Moreover, tooth decay is a very common symptom of excess stomach acid as it wears down the outer layer of your teeth (enamel). As a result, this can lead to excess cavities and weakened teeth. In a recent study, researchers found that over 40% of GERD patients showed significant tooth decay, along with 70% of patients whose reflux had managed to reach the upper esophagus), compared to only 10% of those patients that had no symptoms of reflux. Certainly, reading about the symptoms that accompany stomach acid is disconcerting and worrisome. Nonetheless, being aware of the symptoms and knowing the early signs of their emergence will mitigate the risks of cancer and other chronic ailments like GERD and Barret's esophagus.

So, what can you do about these symptoms and potentially life-altering health concerns if you are experiencing excess stomach acid? Initially, and rather obviously, begin by assessing your diet. If you typically consume large meals, cut down your portions by at least 25%, and avoid eating right before you sleep. The latter is especially important for your digestive track as your body has to work harder to digest food whilst you are asleep and when your body's organs are supposed to be at rest. Also, limit your chocolate and coffee intake. Typically, medical professionals recommend limiting your coffee intake to only 2-3 cups per day at the most. If these levels are exceeded, your body's acidity levels will climb to healthy proportions and heighten your likelihood of acquiring the aforementioned symptoms. In the same way, excess consumption of alcohol and peppermint carry very harmful side-effects. Not mention, smoking is by far the most dangerous to many of your body's organs, especially the esophagus. Taking steps to cut back and eventually quit smoking is strongly recommended to not only avoid esophageal cancer and weakened tooth enamel, but for a bevy of other health-related reasons not directly associated with stomach acidity. When consulting a doctor to address stomach acid symptoms, you will most likely be prescribed an antacid, H2 blocker or a proton pump inhibitor (PPI); all three are available by prescription as well as over the counter.

Where GERD is concerned, there are other major factors that you should look out for. These symptoms are not specific to a particular body type or even certain foods. First, heartburn is, as mentioned, a clear indicator of GERD and is usually an only an occasional issue that is known to affect over 60 million people at least once or twice a month on average. However, for the 20 million individuals who suffer from heartburn on a chronic level through GERD, seemingly unrelated symptoms can inevitably result in numerous other health complications. You are well advised to consult a doctor if you find that you suffer frequent heartburn (two-three times per week regularly).

When you suffer from GERD, acid, food, as well as digestive juices tend to flow back into your esophagus from the pit of your stomach. Over time, this results in esophagitis, thereby leaving the king of the walls of the esophagus extremely vulnerable to additional harm through scarring, tearing and even deterioration. Additionally, while the primary symptom of GERD is heartburn, there are likely to be other symptoms that are far more difficult to diagnose for doctors and patients alike. Notably, doctors refer to a symptom known as, "silent reflux," which includes voice changes, chronic coughing, major and prolonged throat soreness, along with hoarseness. Patients may have a sustained sensation of having a lump in their throatier having the constant urge for having to clear one's throat. Another common symptom of GERD is the effect that stomach acid has on your breathing. Indeed, GERD, for instance, can heighten the extreme effects of asthma and or pneumonia. Whether or not patients have a history of lung problems personally or with regard to their family lineage, GERD can cause difficulty in breathing and persistent shortness of breath. However, treating this particular symptom is especially tricky; according to several recent studies, GERD medication, like PPIs, have been shown to increase pneumonia by directly contributing to the growth of harmful bacteria. Also, researchers have found that many prescribed PPIs suppress coughing that is needed to clear the lungs. As a result, your doctor may be forced to consider the function of your lungs when prescribing PPIs when in the process of treating symptoms associated with acid reflux.

Many people with ulcers from acid reflux tend to spit up blood and or see it in their stool. For a point of clarity, be sure to note that Esophageal ulcers are much different than stomach ulcers as they (stomach) are usually due to bacteria. Blood from esophageal ulcers, however, tend to be red or a darker purple-red color. If you find yourself having such symptoms, be sure to contact your doctor immediately. The immediate response from your doctor will likely be a schedules endoscopy mentioned earlier. In addition, you may also be prescribed acid-blocking or acid-reducing meds can treat these dangerous stomach ulcer.

An overarching common symptom of acid reflux is a lower quality of life. According to a 2004 study from Europe, whereby 6,000 GERD patients reported that their quality of life had been significantly diminished due to problems that are associated with drink, food and sleep, along with social and physical limitations. Not to mention, there can be major financial implications from having to buy an abundant amount of medications to treat the myriad symptoms of acid reflux, as well as the possible surgical procedures and endoscopy sessions that may be needed if the symptoms escalate to advanced stages. Moreover, the quality of life for patients of GERD was strikingly similar to heart-attack patients and was even lower, in certain cases, for those patients struggling with diabetes and cancer.

Generally, the healing time-frame for GERD is around 2 to 8 weeks. If allowed to persist without medicinal intervention, symptoms of GERD can inflict a considerable amount of damage. For example, reflux esophagitis (RO) can create visible and painful cracks and breaks in the esophageal mucosa. In order to fully and effectively heal RO, acid suppression for a prolonged period (roughly 3-9 weeks) is required and will likely be the timeframe advised by your doctor. Keep in mind that healing rates will rapidly improve as acid suppression increases.

Chronic stress is also a significant factor in the development, growth and. persistence of acid reflux. Our digestive system, moreover, is intricately associated with our nervous system. When stress presents itself, especially in an overwhelming or uncontrollable manner, our digestive system will then receive a lower amount of blood flow, thus causing various issues. Further, our gut bacteria are implicated in our management of stress at increasing levels, so probiotics are helpful in helping the management of this development.

Chapter 2: The role of Fibre, Prebiotics and Probiotics

Incorporating key changes into your diet can carry massive benefits with regard to dealing with the many symptoms of acid reflux. Specifically, consuming more fiber is an excellent way to mitigate the harsh symptoms. An important point of clarity is the distinction between dietary fiber, defined as edible but non-digestible carbohydrate-based material, and insoluble fiber. Dietary fiber is mainly available in abundance naturally in many cereals, grains, plants, and vegetables as these all play a major role in gastrointestinal health. Given the importance of fiber, and its positive impact in easing the symptoms of acid reflux, many people on average are dangerously deficient in fiber. This deficiency includes both the soluble and insoluble forms of fiber. The main difference between these two forms of fiber are found in their role in digestion; insoluble fiber expedites the travel of foods through the gastrointestinal tract, while solute fibers have been shown to slow the digestion process.

While the varied and, at times, monotonous science concerning acid reflux is still in progress and remains to be settled. Nevertheless, the theoretical benefits of adequate intake of fiber include avoiding trigger foods altogether, as well as the stomach-filling "full" effect of fiber and fewer relaxation reactions of the anti-reflux valve residing between the stomach and the esophagus. Even still, there exists a persistent relationship between acid reflux trigger and the role of fiber. To elaborate, soluble fiber has been shown to induce the body to draw fluid out of already digested food, which then contributes added bulk to your meals which leaves you with a feeling of being "full" for a far more prolonged period of time. As it is commonly found within such sources as barley, peas as well as oat bran, soluble fiber does play an active role in regulating glucose levels and may even contribute to signaling the brain that the stomach is in fact full both during and after eating a meal of any size. Moreover, smaller meals can help acid reflux by refraining from overfilling your stomach. Whereas, insoluble fiber as found within vegetables and whole grains can speed up the passage of stomach contents to your intestinal tract, thereby decreasing your body's propensity for reflux.

Additionally, fatty, fried foods are typically much lower in fiber and are also frequently accompanied by the triggering symptoms of regurgitation, indigestion, and heartburn. Indeed, a fiber-rich diet like fresh fruits, vegetables, and whole-grain bread can tend to contribute to fewer instances of reflux symptoms arising. Some dietary fibers are also widely considered to be probiotics. Note the key distinction between prebiotics and probiotics: the latter refers to the specific helpful bacteria itself, with prebiotic referring to bacterial nutrients. In other words, prebiotics are nutrients which are left for bacteria to digest, or, more plainly, fuel to encourage the balanced bacterial growth within digestive organs. Here, the role of fiber in greatly improving the many symptoms of acid reflux is illuminated; this role is as a bacterial intermediary. On the whole, nonetheless, particular items in your diet tend to perform a seemingly minor role in the symptoms associated with acid reflux. Those who suffer from chronic acid reflux are strongly advised to avoid those specific foods that can aggravate painful heartburn and regurgitation; however, eliminating a broad range of food from your diet is no recommenced as it can detrimental to your overall health. Instead, you should note foods and beverages that can trigger acid reflux specifically and root them out from your diet as soon as possible.

There is a tremendous amount of evidence in favor of incorporating a fiber-rich diet into your daily routine. Notably, the benefits are particular to the overall maintenance of your gut and with regard to managing the amount of harmful bacteria native to that region of your body. A study from 2004 that involved over 65,000 people revealed that fiber intake was associated with the improved perception of acid reflux symptoms. Also, this study revealed people who consumed high fiber bread were nearly three times as likely to experience relief of acid reflux symptoms compared to people who consumed bread with lower fiber content. Granted, the reasons for these results remains unknown; however, the authors of the broad study have speculated that the digestive process of fiber can also be a catalyst for enhanced muscle relaxation from the stomach through the esophagus as it tightens the anti-reflux valve.

So, what are the disadvantages of fiber in acid reflux? It is true that fiber is especially helpful when serving to ease acid reflux symptoms, excess fiber consumption has been shown to aggravate the symptoms. A study published in a medical journalism 2014 indicated that consuming a minimum of 10 grams of highly fermentable starches each day can significantly contribute to painful episodes of acid reflux symptoms. An additional study noted that nine participants who were diagnosed with GERD, those patients who consumed a prebiotic known as fructooligo also had elevated instances of acid reflux symptoms than those patients who were given a placebo.

There are many aspects to consider when striving to efficiently manage acid reflux symptoms. Among them, dietary fiber is perhaps the most important or, at the very least, the most consequential. For instance, while being excessively overweight is certainly risk factor as far as GERD is concerned, adequate consumption of healthy fiber will aid in keeping the weight at a healthy level. Excess fiber, however, causes stomach distension in may people, along with enhanced stomach pressure as well as prolonged emptying on the stomach in many cases, all of which have shown to lead to accentuated acid reflux symptoms. Medical professionals specializing in gastroenterology strongly recommend implementing lifestyle changes such as eating smaller sized meals on a frequent basis (as opposed to larger meals a few times per day), limiting overall consumption of carbonated beverages and foods high in salt content with the intent of improving the acid reflux symptoms. Note that women over the age of 50 should try to consume 25 grams per day; on the other hand, men under 50 are strongly advised to consume 38 grams of fiber each day. While consuming more laxatives is often the approach undertaken by people dealing with symptoms of acid reflux, medical professionals advise increasing your fiber content within your diet for maximized results, as well as maintaining your overall health as laxatives can take a substantial toll on your body and its digestive tract. Consuming a higher amount of fiber will strengthen your stool, keep wastes traveling more smoothly through your intestinal tract, along with preventing constipation. During this process of consuming more fibre, be sure to also ensure that you are consuming plenty of water as well; for fiber to have its absolute best effect, it is imperative that your body remain as hydrated as possible to make sure that waste moves smoothly along your intestinal tract rather than building up due to rigidity.

A good source of probiotics and fiber is yogurt, which carries "good" bacteria helpful for overall maintenance of gut health. A healthy gut is paramount for an efficient and well-functioning intestinal tract and digestive system. Prebiotics and probiotics are, essentially, analogous to food for the bacteria in your stomach; bananas, corn, and whole wheat are additional food sources that are high in prebiotics. Moreover, one of the most beneficial aspects of a fiber-rich diet is the notion that high-fiber foods help control your cravings for snacks. Certainly, high fiber diets can help you lose weight as it displaces other calories for overall maintenance of health.

Guarding against illness, fiber-rich diets will also lower your chances of developing major gut-related illnesses such as diverticulitis. This condition, pockets in the walls of colon trap waste as opposed to moving it along. While doctors remain unsure of the direct catalyst(s) for the illness, consuming a high-fiber diet moves waste fervently along through your system. Along with diverticulitis, a high-fiber diet also eases and prevents irritable bowel syndrome— which has also been linked to acid reflux, albeit a rarer, more extreme symptom. Nevertheless, the most common symptom of acid reflux— heartburn— is quelled by a fiber-rich diet.

Probiotics are becoming increasingly linked to the management of the symptoms associated with acid reflux and alleviating these issues. For a more technical explanation, as we are already aware that probiotics are an effective way of balancing the gut bacteria inside of our bodies, they also help combat against a bacterial infection knows as, H. pylori. This bacterial infection usually originates in childhood. This bacteria, found in the stomach, can alter the environment around them through reducing the acidity levels so that they can survive for longer periods of time. By penetrating the lining of the stomach, thereby remaining hidden and protected by the mucous membrane so that the body's immune defenses cannot reach them. In addition, these bacteria tend to secrete an enzyme called urease, which converts urea to ammonia. The presence of ammonia in this instance is significant because it reduces the stomach acidity around the specific area where the bacteria is found. Coincidentally, it is this lower stomach acid that is often mistaken— by doctors and patients alike— for acid reflux. Can probiotics help combat H. pylori? Well, many medical researchers believe that probiotics can, in fact, help battle this bacteria in several key ways. For one, probiotics are believed to strengthen the protective barrier against H. pylori by producing antimicrobial substances, along with competing against H. pylori for what is known as adhesion receptors (space on the lining of the stomach). Also, it is believed that probiotics assist in stabilizing the gut's mucosal barrier. Many researchers even argue that the production of relatively large amounts of lactate is another inhibitory factor of H. pylori due to the possibility that it could lower the H. pylori urease. Not to mention, probiotics may also be effective in modifying inflammation levels by interacting with the epithelial cells that are responsible for managing the secretion of inflammatory proteins in the gut.

Depending on the particular cause of your acid reflux, probiotics can be incredibly useful for alleviating the painful symptoms. Probiotics can be taken in conjunction with an antacid without worry of the antacid overtaking the positive benefits of the probiotic. More importantly, your approach should be to uncover the root of your acid reflux and adjust medical intervention accordingly. Of course, you doctor plays a huge role in this process, especially in diagnosing the specific cause of your acid reflux; still, it is your responsibility to seek medical expertise so that you can tackle the root of the symptoms as opposed to addressing the individual symptoms as they arise. Being aware of the triggers in both the food and drinks that you consume, managing your stress levels regardless of how often they fluctuate, and finding the specific levels of acid within your stomach are critical steps to address the symptoms of acid reflux. More likely than not, the best method of dealing with your symptoms will be to implement a diverse approach that incorporates a range of approaches rather than relying solely on medical intervention.

Chapter 3: Understanding the role of proteins, carbs, AND fats in healing acid damage

In recent years, there have been increasing reports concerning the benefits of a low-carb diet in healing the damage induced by acid damage. This may seem counterintuitive given the notion that the standard treatment for GERD includes the removal of certain foods that increase acidity in the stomach, for example, tomato sauces which are believed to be contributing causes of excess stomach acidity. Also, as mentioned in chapter 1, the removal of coffee, alcohol, smoking, and peppermint are other dietary and lifestyle changes that ease GERD symptoms. Additionally, researchers have found that diets with a higher amount of carbohydrates can significantly elevate symptoms of acid reflux. Whereas, a low-carb diet has also been shown to reduce symptoms of GERD. While many health researchers and medical experts have expressed concern over the exceptionally low proportion of daily calories from fat and protein in low-carb diets, as wells calorie levels being considerably lower in these diet than recommended. Nevertheless, the effects of gastroesophageal reflux disease have been shown to be significantly reduced after implementation of a low-carb diet. For a case in point, following a 2001 research study in which 5 individuals with diverse ranges of GERD symptoms and across the age spectrum, engaged in a low-carb diet, each of the 5 research participants showed significant relief of symptoms. Granted, throughout the duration of the study, which spanned 8 months, 3 of the 5 research participants also reduced their coffee intake concurrently.

The concurrent reduction of coffee, coupled with lower intake of carbohydrates, was shown to be effective in reducing symptoms such as heartburn and stomach pain. Interestingly, while coffee reduction was a contributing factor, observations from a few of the participants revealed that exacerbating foods such as coffee and fat are less pertinent when a low-carb diet is strictly followed. In other words, when implementing a low-carb diet, the effects of classic factors like coffee and fat intake are vastly diminished even if their consumption is not significantly reduced. So, whether or not you choose to reduce coffee and fat intake significantly, you are likely to reduce most GERD symptoms by solely undertaking a low-carb diet. Therefore, the logical conclusion to draw from these findings is that a low-carb diet is a significant factor for reducing the symptoms of acid reflux. This conclusion gains even more credibility when considering the propensity for high-carb diets to aggravate GERD symptoms.

In addition to lower carbohydrates, lean sources of protein and healthy fats are beneficial for reducing symptoms associated with acid reflux. Lean proteins found in eggs are a great addition to your diet for reducing acid reflux symptoms; however, they are a problem for many people due to elevated cholesterol. If eggs are an issue for you, be sure to consume only egg whites and refrain for consuming higher fat yolks—which have been shown to elevate GERD symptoms. Moreover, as high-fat meals and fried food typically descries LES pressure thereby delaying emptying of the stomach and boosting the risk of acid reflux, it is in your best interest to choose lean grilled meats, as well as poached, baked or broiled meats. Boosting proteins, in the way, will also provide benefits for your overall health as well. Also, complex carbohydrates, as found in rice, whole grain bread, couscous and oatmeal carry excellent benefits for reducing GERD symptoms and easing any scarring that may already be present in the walls of your esophagus. Specifically, brown rice and whole grains add valuable fiber your diet. Root vegetables such as potatoes are excellent sources of healthy carbohydrates and easily digestible fiber. Remember to refrain from incorporating too much garlic and onion while preparing your meals, which are can commonly irritate the esophagus and stomach lining.

Along with proteins and complex carbs, incorporating healthy fats has great benefits for easing GERD symptoms and other symptoms accompanying acid reflux. A type of nutrient, fat is high in calories but certainly a necessary component of your diet. Keep in mind, however, fats can vary and they do not all have the same effect on your body. On the whole, you are well advised to avoid consuming a high amount of saturated fats as typically found in dairy and meat, along with trans fats found in processed foods, shortening and margarine. As a replacement, unsaturated fats from fish and or plants are recommended; some examples of monounsaturated fats include sesame, olive, canola, sunflower, peanuts, seeds and nuts, as well as butter. In addition, examples of polyunsaturated fats include such oils as safflower, corn, flaxseed and walnut, fatty fish such as salmon and trout, along with soybean.

Some other helpful tips for reducing acid reflux symptoms include chewing gum, as long as it is not spearmint- or peppermint-flavored. Chewing gum increases the amount of saliva production in your mouth and also reduces the amount of acid in your esophagus. While alcohol consumption has already been mentioned in earlier chapters, research suggests that some people begin to experience extreme symptoms after only one drink; if you fall into this category, be sure to experiment with your levels to uncover what amount is best for you. Additionally, during and after each meal, particularly bigger meals, be sure to remain aware of your posture. Generally, it is a good idea to sit up while you are eating and avoid lying flat on your back for at least hours post-meal. Standing up and walking around the room after a big meal can help encourage the flow of gastric juices in the right direction. Further, avoiding eating big meals before bed can help you refrain from overloading your digestive system while you sleep. Digestion increases the overall amount of gastric acid that is present within your stomach. When laying down, LES's ability to inhibit stomach contents from traveling through the esophagus decreases significantly. When operating concurrently, excess stomach acid and remaining in a reclined position for an unexpended period of time create an abundance of acid reflux symptoms. On the whole, consuming a large meal for less than 3 to 4 hours prior to bed is generally not advisable for those suffering from persistent GERD symptoms; however, the timing of these symptoms can certainly vary depending on the individual.

In a 2017 research study on the benefits of healthy dietary changes versus drug intervention, researchers studied the effects of dietary changes to a type of reflux known as laryngopharyngeal reflux or LPR. This reflux is essentially triggered when pepsin, a digestive enzyme from the stomach, reaches the sensitive tissues in the upper section of the digestive tract. Symptoms like throat clearing and hoarseness are common with pepsin in the throat and or upper part of the digestive tract. In the study, the researchers had participants suffering from acid reflux switch to a Mediterranean diet and consuming significantly more water, thereby neutralizing excess acid. In this particular study, participants avoided classic triggers such as coffee, peppermint, alcohol, fatty and spicy foods, chocolate and soda. Another set of participants were given pharmaceutical drugs to ease GERD symptoms.

After a six week timeframe, participants of the study reported a greater percent of declines in their GERD symptoms as those participants that had used drugs to address the symptoms. Granted, the study did not elaborate on the particular ways in which that the diet and increased water consumption eased the symptoms; nonetheless, the Mediterranean diet incorporates eating mostly plant-based fruits and vegetables. In addition, the increased water can mitigate pepsin's acidity levels in the throat. As mentioned, fruits, vegetables and water are great methods of reducing acid reflux and GERD symptoms. With this in mind, the positive benefits experienced by the study's participants is not surprising in the least.

Adjusting your diet for GERD does not require removing all of the foods that you typically enjoy eating. Instead, a few simple changes to your diet if more than enough to address the uncomfortable symptoms of GERD. Your aim in addressing the GERD symptoms should be to create a well-rounded, nutrient-based diet that incorporates a variety of foods that include vegetables, fruits, complex carbs, healthy fats and lean sources of protein. Healing acid reflux damage is made significantly easier when starting with dietary changes that add healthy and diverse foods. Coupled with medical intervention (if required), healthy dietary changes can carry great benefits for healing scarring in your esophagus and stomach, as well as symptoms such as heartburn, bloating and even tooth decay.

Chapter 4: Exercise to reduce acid reflux

When GERD symptoms escalate and you are still in the early stages of implementing dietary changes to address acid reflux symptoms, exercise can be a great option for reducing the symptoms. When GERD symptoms begin to arise, high-impact physical activities like running, skipping rope and jumping exercises. If you are overweight or obese, a weight loss of 10% has been shown to reduce GERD symptoms like heartburn, bloating and reflux. A self-reported analysis study of individuals experiencing GERD symptoms fund that those who reduced their Body Mass Index (BMI) by 2 kilograms or 4.4 pounds or more, along with the circumference of their waist by 5cm or more has improved their GERD symptoms significantly. In contrast, there are also certain exercises that can induce reflux by opening the lower esophageal sphincter (LES) during workouts such as heavy lifting, stomach crunches, or other high impact exercises. When the LES opens, stomach acid travels up into the esophagus causing heartburn.

There are some common sense tips concerning exercise for managing GERD symptoms. First, this twice about how much and what you are eating prior to starting your exercise routine. Obviously, less food in your stomach is ideal. If you are too full, you should wait at least 1 to 2 hours before initiating your exercise routine. This will allow for food to pass fro your stomach through to the small intestine. With less food in your stomach while exercising, it is significantly less likely that you will experience the painful and annoying symptoms of acid reflux such as heartburn and bloating. Next, you should choose the food you consume with thought and, in some instances, caution. Generally, you should avoid foods that trigger GERD symptoms (choosing complex carbohydrates is advised). Your stomach does metabolize these foods much faster than others through a process known as gastric emptying. Moreover, diabetics should avoid high fat and high protein foods before exercise due to being more susceptible to experiencing slow gastric emptying. Experts also suggest adjusting your workout if you suffer from frequent GERD symptoms. Starting at a slower pace with workouts that put less strain on your body like controlled walking and controlled weight training in either a sitting or standing position is strongly recommended. Whereas, high impact, high-intensity workouts like running, rowing and cycling and induce acid reflux. Additionally, acrobatic workouts and gymnastics can also disrupt stomach contents. The key is to avoid exercises that jostle the LES and reflux, these are typically positions that put your body in awkward positions like being upside down defying gravity in one way or another.

A great exercise that carries tremendous benefits for improving and relieving acid reflux symptoms and digestion is yoga. One particular study from 2014 found that six months of yoga significantly reduced acid reflux and stomach bloating, along with improved esophagitis. Again, however, try to avoid positions that heighten GERD symptoms. If any of these "lifestyle" changes fail to improve your GERD symptoms during exercise, be sure to consult your doctor about being prescribed medication for acid-suppression. And, of course, engaging in a constant exercise routine is not only very beneficial with regard to improving your GERD symptoms, but also for the maintenance of your overall health.

Chapter 5: How to live a reflux free life?

As you may have already noticed, acid reflex can be induced by an abundance of factors ranging from diet, bad habits, poor sleep hygiene, and many other factors. Clearly, it isn't just as simple as cutting out bad habits and instilling a series of great dietary and lifestyle changes. But whether you are able to successfully implement these changes or not does not, thankfully, hinge on strict adherence to a stringent diet or eliminating some of your favorite guilty habits. But before you can begin to consider stepping into a reflux-free life, you should be cognizant of the stages of reflux and recovery.

Firstly, almost everyone who suffers from GERD begins with normal LES and little to no reflux. The severity level of GERD, therefore, more than likely correlates to best with the overall degree of damage inflicted upon the sphincter. Note, however, that this is not easy to determine. Normally, the amount of damage to your sphincter correlates with the overall severity of acid reflux symptoms. This severity is most often determined by the volume, frequency, and duration of reflux episodes. In turn, these factors will correlate with GERD symptoms such as regurgitation and heartburn. If you are diagnosed with GERD, your strategy for addressing the symptoms and eventually overcoming them should first be to containment. Unfortunately, damage to your LES caused by GERD cannot be reversed by drugs and is permanent. Nonetheless, many patients of GERD have been able to live with these symptoms and with functionality despite damage to the sphincter. Changing simple lifestyle habits, such as sleeping and eating, can significantly decrease and prevent severe reflux episodes in spite of damage to your sphincter.

In Stage 1 of GERD, known as Mild GERD, most adults currently have minimal damage to their LES and tend to experience mild GERD occasionally. Most often, the adults are left with either tolerating occasional heartburn or will have to use over-the-counter acid suppressive medications from the onset of symptoms through its subsequent stages. Typically, when taking drugs to address the symptoms, quality of life for patients is not affected because the medications are very effective in suppressing symptoms. If you choose to take medication to address symptoms, make sure that you are also cleaning up your diet. If you continue to consume trigger foods and beverages, like coffee and certain sauces, for example, the benefits you garner from medication will be minimal and your recovery will be prolonged if not inhibited altogether. Replacing these meals with smaller, leaner meals that do not pose a threat to inducing symptoms of GERD is recommended. This will ease heartburn and lessen the damage to your sphincter.

In stage 2, known as Moderate GERD, symptoms are far more difficult to control and use of prescribed acid-suppressive drugs will be needed. In this stage, reflux is accompanied by symptoms that are far more intense than stage 1. Therefore, medicinal intervention is needed to mitigate the damage and pain caused by these symptoms. Still, many symptoms in this stage can be managed by using acid-suppressive drugs for prolonged periods of time. Keep in mind that over-the-counter medication can provide insufficient relief; whereas, prescription strength medications are needed in order for you to manage GERD symptoms effectively. Additionally, stage 3, or, Severe GERD, can result in a very low quality if life and is generally considered to be an extremely serious problem by medical professionals specializing in GERD. Because prescription grade acid-suppressive drugs and medicinal intervention usually do not control symptoms, regurgitation is frequent. In Stage 3, it is entirely possible that complications associated with erosive GERD are present. Lastly, stage 4, or, reflux-induced esophageal cancer, is quite obviously the most serious stage. The result of numerous years of severe reflux, nearly 16% of all long-term reflux sufferers progress to this extremely advanced stage. Due to the long-term reflux, the esophagus' lining has been heavily damaged, thereby resulting in a high degree of cellular changes. Also, stage 4 is the stage that involves the pre-cancerous condition called Barrett's esophagus and or an even more severe condition called dysplasia. Granted, these conditions are not cancerous. However, they are capable of raising the risk of developing reflux-induced esophageal cancer. Accordingly, at this stage, common GERD symptoms are likely to also be accompanied by a strong burning sensation in the throat, chronic coughing, and persistent hoarseness. A narrowing of the esophagus, or strictures, will also be present in this stage, and can also be characterized by the sensation that food is sticking to your throat. However, this is only a feeling associated with strictures. Notably, this symptom is also caused by esophageal cancer. Keep in mind that stage 4 GERD can only be diagnosed by a medical professional through an endoscopy and from an intrusive biopsy of cells retrieved from the lower esophagus.

A 30-day recovery plan for GERD symptom can be easily broken into weekly steps. In the first week, you will presumably be trying to lean off of the medication that you have been prescribed. A reversion plan of this nature should take into account a variety of approaches that incorporate dietary changes, exercise routines, sleep schedules, and other lifestyle changes. Drinking more tea and water is strongly recommended throughout your 30-day reversion plan, as long as the tea is not peppermint-flavored. Also, in your first week of recovery, be sure to get as much sleep as possible, in conjunction with eating 2 to 3 hours before you sleep. A meal should also be incorporated throughout this entire 30-day stretch. This plan should include egg whites in the morning, instead of coffee switch to tea for your caffeine fix. For lunch, whole grain bread with lean meat- chicken or turkey preferably- with light sauce and a bevy of vegetables. Moreover, dinner should include a balanced meal that provides nutrients and foods that will not induce heartburn. Remember, this meal should be consumed a few hours before bed so that your body has time to properly digest the food. Also, be sure to refrain from lying directly on your back after your meal; as mentioned, this will induce acid reflux symptoms like heartburn and excess bloating.

In week 2, in keeping with the consumption of nutrient-rich food and water consumption from the previous week, you should begin an exercise routine of you have been devoid of routine prior to week 2. A consistent exercise routine will help maintain overall health so that your body has excess strength and energy to overcome the wear and damage inflicted from GERD symptoms. Also, a consistent exercise routine will boost your metabolism so that you can burn off excess unhealthy fats and complex carbohydrates that can cause strain to your body and induce reflux symptoms. In the third week of your 30-day revision plan, you can slightly increase the size of your meals. Still, make sure that the overall size of your meals remain relatively small, with only slight additions where you may see fit. By week three, your exercise routine, water consumption, and sleep habits should be starting to feel more routine and many of reflux your symptoms will begin to diminish. Moreover, leading into week 4, your diet should continue to incorporate nuts, vegetables, fruits, tea, and other plant-based foods and drinks to expedite the healing process. However, the final week of your 30-day recovery plan is vital for sustaining the progress that you have presumably made since the start of the month. It is vital because you must ensure that you do not get too comfortable in your routine that you allow for gradual decline back into the habits that spawned your acid reflux. Pushing through this final week will augment your progress and solidify your path to living a reflux-free life. Specifically, with regard to your diet, you can incorporate the following fruit and vegetable smoothie recipe. Smoothies and healthy shakes are an excellent meal replacement option for optimal health and recovery from acid reflux.

1. Add 2 scoops of frozen berries into a 400ml cup

2. Add 2 scoops of spinach from a 250ml scoop

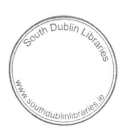

3. Add 2 tablespoons of Chia Seeds

4. Add 2 tablespoons of hemp hearts

5. Add 1 tablespoon of peanut butter

This smoothie should be blended with water to ensure that it is not excessively thick.